NEW YORK REVIEW BOOKS
CLASSICS

FIGHTING FOR LIFE

SARA JOSEPHINE BAKER (1873–1945) was born in Pough-keepsie, New York, and attended the Woman's Medical College of the New York Infirmary. As the first director of New York's Bureau of Child Hygiene from 1908 to 1923, Baker's work with poor mothers and children in the immigrant communities of New York City dramatically reduced maternal and child mortality and became a model for cities across the country. On two occasions she helped to track down Mary Mallon, the cook who came to be known as Typhoid Mary. Baker wrote fifty journal articles and more than two hundred pieces for the popular press about preventive medicine, as well as six books: *Healthy Babies, Healthy Mothers, Healthy Children* (all 1920), *The Growing Child* (1923), *Child Hygiene* (1925), and her autobiography, *Fighting for Life* (1939). In the 1930s Baker, along with her partner of many years, the novelist Ida Wylie, and their friend Dr. Louise Pearce, moved to a two-hundred-year-old farm in New Jersey, where she lived until her death.

HELEN EPSTEIN is a writer specializing in public health and an adjunct professor at Bard College. She has advised numerous organizations, including the United States Agency for International Development, the World Bank, Human Rights Watch, and UNICEF. She is the author of *Th*
Losing the Fight Against AIDS i
articles to many publications, inc
Books and *The New York Times M*

FIGHTING FOR LIFE

S. JOSEPHINE BAKER

Introduction by
HELEN EPSTEIN

NEW YORK REVIEW BOOKS

New York

THIS IS A NEW YORK REVIEW BOOK
PUBLISHED BY THE NEW YORK REVIEW OF BOOKS
435 Hudson Street, New York, NY 10014
www.nyrb.com

Library of Congress Cataloging-in-Publication Data
Baker, S. Josephine (Sara Josephine), 1873–1945, author.
Fighting for life / by S. Josephine Baker ; introduction by Helen Epstein.
    p. ; cm. — (New York review books classics)
Includes index.
Reprint of: Baker, S. Josephine (Sara Josephine), 1873–1945. Fighting for life.
New York : The Macmillan Company, 1939. 264 p.
ISBN 978-1-59017-706-8 (paperback : alk. paper)
I. Title. II. Series: New York Review Books classics.
[DNLM: 1. Baker, S. Josephine (Sara Josephine), 1873–1945. 2. Physicians—
New York City—Autobiography. 3. Child Mortality—history—New York
City. 4. Child Welfare—history—New York City. 5. History, 19th Century—
New York City. 6. History, 20th Century—New York City. 7. Public Health—
history—New York City. WZ 100]
R690
610.92—dc23
[B]

                            2013020026

ISBN 978-1-59017-706-8
Available as an electronic book; ISBN 978-1-59017-707-5

Printed in the United States of America on acid-free paper.
10 9 8 7 6 5 4 3 2 1

INTRODUCTION

The Lower East Side of New York was one of the most densely populated square miles on the face of the earth in the 1890s. The photo-essayist Jacob Riis famously described it as a world of bad smells, scooting rats, ash barrels, dead goats, and little boys drinking beer out of milk cartons. Six thousand people might be packed into a single city block, many in tenements with sanitary facilities so foul as to repel anyone who dared approach. City health inspectors called the neighborhood "the suicide ward"; one tenement was referred to—in an official New York City Health Department report, no less—as an "out and out hog pen."[*]

Diarrhea epidemics blazed through the slums each summer, killing thousands of children every week. In the sweatshops of what was then known as "Jewtown," children with smallpox and typhus dozed in heaps of garments destined for fashionable Broadway shops. Desperate mothers paced the streets trying to soothe their feverish children, and white mourning cloths hung from every story of every building. A third of the children born in the slums died before their fifth birthday.

In the European farming villages where many of these immigrants came from, people spent most of their time outdoors in the fresh air and sunshine and seldom encountered more than a few hundred people in the course of lifetime. "Crowd diseases"—

---

[*]Oscar Handlin, *The Uprooted: The Epic Story of the Great Migrations That Made the American People* (University of Pennsylvania Press, 2002).

measles, dysentery, typhoid, diphtheria, trachoma, and so on—
were rare, and the immigrants had little idea of how to prevent
them. Some parents vainly tried to administer folk remedies; others just prepared the little funeral shrouds in silence.

It was in the 1890s that Sara Josephine Baker decided to become
a doctor. Not the Josephine Baker who would become celebrated as
a cabaret star and dance at the Folies Bergère in a banana miniskirt
but the New York City public health official in a shirtwaist and
four-in-hand necktie, her short hair parted in the middle like Theodore Roosevelt, whom she admired. By the time Baker retired from
the New York City Health Department in 1923, she was
famous across the nation for saving the lives of ninety thousand
inner-city children. The public health measures she implemented,
many still in use today, have saved the lives of millions more world-
wide. She was also a charming, funny storyteller, and her remarkable memoir, *Fighting for Life*, is an honest, unsentimental, and
deeply compassionate account of how one American woman helped
launch a public health revolution.

Baker grew up in a modestly prosperous Poughkeepsie family
and studied medicine at the Women's Medical College in Manhattan, which was run by Emily Blackwell, the sister of the more
famous Elizabeth, America's first woman doctor. Baker graduated
second in her class. The only course she failed was The Normal
Child, taught by Dr. Annie Sturges Daniel, a pioneer health
educator who also campaigned for better housing conditions for
the poor. Baker had to retake the class and in studying for it
became fascinated with "that little pest, the normal child" whom
she would go on to make the focus of her career.

After graduation, Baker took an internship at the New England
Hospital for Women and Children in Boston and then returned to
establish a private practice in New York. She once examined the
actress Lillian Russell, but most of her patients resided in the tin

squatters' shacks of Amsterdam Avenue and couldn't pay her. In need of money, she applied for a job with the Department of Health and was hired in 1902.

Medicine in those days required a certain daring. While still in Boston, she almost killed a drunk who was beating his pregnant wife as Baker was trying to deliver their baby. As a New York City health inspector, she administered smallpox injections to snoozing hoboes in Bowery flophouses, fielded calls from Tammany politicians requesting that she hire their cast-off mistresses as nurses (she declined), and chased down the notorious cook Typhoid Mary through the streets of Manhattan. Baker had to sit on Mary all the way to the hospital to keep her in the ambulance.

Modern readers might be put off by Baker's tendency—common in those days—to generalize about the various ethnic groups she encountered in the city's variegated slums. Blacks come off well; the Irish all seem to have been slapstick drunks. However, she clearly understood that their misery and dissolution were part of a wider culture of official corruption and indifference to the poor, which afflicted even her own Health Department.

In the tenements of Hell's Kitchen, Baker "climbed stair after stair, knocked on door after door, met drunk after drunk, filthy mother after filthy mother and dying baby after dying baby." Most of her fellow health inspectors didn't bother to make rounds at all; they just forged their records and went on their way. Baker, who might well have been fired for making everyone else look bad, was lucky to have the support of the Tammany-affiliated but nevertheless reform-inclined mayor George McClellan, elected in 1903. He appointed a new health commissioner who dismissed the other inspectors and promoted Baker. In 1908, she was put in charge of the Health Department's new Bureau of Child Hygiene, the first of its kind in the country.

There she changed the way we think about public health. Until then, the Health Department had sought to track down sick children and refer them to physicians, a mostly futile endeavor in the absence of antibiotics and other tools of modern medicine. Baker decided that the new bureau's mission would instead be prevention. The city had an established and efficient system of birth registration. As soon as a child was born, her name and address were reported to the Health Department. Baker reasoned that if every new mother were properly taught how to feed and care for a baby and recognize the signs of illness, the mother would have a much better chance of keeping the child alive.

In her first year at the Bureau of Child Hygiene, Baker sent nurses to the most deadly ward on the Lower East Side. They were to visit every new mother within a day of delivery, encouraging exclusive breast-feeding, fresh air, and regular bathing, and discouraging hazardous practices such as feeding the baby beer or allowing him to play in the gutter. This advice was entirely conventional, but the results were extraordinary: That summer, 1,200 fewer children died in that district compared to the previous year; elsewhere in the city the death rate remained high. The home-visiting program was soon implemented citywide, and in 1910, a network of "milk stations" staffed by nurses and doctors began offering regular baby examinations and safe formula for older infants and the infants of women who couldn't breast-feed. In just three years, the infant death rate in New York City fell by 40 percent, and in December 1911, *The New York Times* hailed the city as the healthiest in the world.

Articles about Baker's lifesaving campaigns appeared in newspapers from Oklahoma to Michigan to California. In the late 1910s, she and other reformers drafted a bill to create a nationwide network of home-visiting programs and maternal and child health clinics modeled on the programs in New York. But the American Medical Association—backed by powerful Republicans averse to spending money on the poor—claimed the program was tantamount to Bolshevism. Baker was in Washington the day a young New England doctor explained the AMA's position to a congressional committee:

> "We oppose this Bill because, if you are going to save the lives of all these women and children at public expense, what inducement will there be for young men to study medicine?" Senator Sheppard, the chairman, stiffened and leaned forward: "Perhaps I didn't understand you correctly," he said; "You surely don't mean you want women and children to die unnecessarily or live in constant danger of sickness so there will be something for young doctors to do?" "Why not?" said the New England doctor, who did at least have the courage to admit the issue; "That's the will of God, isn't it?"

Baker's public health innovations were numerous. In addition to the home-visiting programs and community baby clinics, she established the position of the school nurse, developed special capsules for delivering silver nitrate to the eyes of newborns to prevent blindness due to congenital gonorrhea, invented a window board for improving ventilation in houses, and created a more efficient method of medical record keeping. She even designed a set of baby clothes that was more convenient and comfortable than the swaddling traditionally used in the immigrant ghettos.

The massive declines in child mortality that Baker helped bring about are frequently attributed to improved nutrition and a general improvement in working and living conditions, and to the availability of vaccines and antibiotics. However, demographers who have studied this subject in detail have concluded that it had little to do with any of these things. Most vaccines and antibiotics weren't available until after World War II and the "general uplift" in nutrition and living conditions occurred at the end of the nineteenth century, decades before the mortality decline. This may have set the stage for the drop in the death rate that followed, but the survival of babies didn't substantially improve until safer milk supplies became widely available and, even more crucially, campaigns like Baker's had helped women understand germs and how to avoid them, so they could provide better care for their children.*

But safe milk and hygiene aren't the only things children need to survive. Baker was the first to prove scientifically that they also need love. In an era when reliable birth control was unavailable and abortion was unsafe and illegal, hundreds of newborns were abandoned each year in New York City. Babies turned up in parks and alleyways or on the doorsteps of fashionable houses. These foundlings were assumed to be illegitimate and until 1870 weren't even welcome at Catholic charity orphanages. Most ended up in squalid municipal almshouses with the paupers, drunks, and insane; nearly all of them died. But in 1915, a foundling hospital opened on Randall's Island under the direction of Baker's Bureau of Child Hygiene. There trained nurses provided the babies with state-of-the-art care and feeding. Nonetheless, close to half of them still died. In what Baker's nurses referred to as the "hopeless ward," where the most premature, sickly babies lay in tiny boxes lined with cotton wool, virtually none survived.

At the time, many doctors would have been unconcerned about this. While the deaths of older infants and children might be at-

---

*Samuel Preston and Michael Haines, *Fatal Years: Child Mortality in Late Nineteenth-Century America* (Princeton University Press, 1991), chapter 6.

tributed to inadequate hygiene and nutrition and prevented accordingly, eugenically minded child health experts believed that the deaths of newborns, defined as children aged under a month or so, were due to their inborn "sub-normality"; there was nothing doctors could do for them. For the benefit of racial hygiene, it was probably better not to care for them. After all, they'd only grow up and pass their sickly genes on to the next generation.

But Baker didn't agree that the fate of these infants was inevitable. She had noticed that though infant mortality had plummeted in the slums due to the bureau's efforts, it hadn't budged in wealthier neighborhoods. "Sometimes," she writes, "it really looked as if a baby born in a dingy tenement room had a better chance to survive its first year, given reasonable care, than a baby born with a silver spoon in its mouth and taken care of by a trained nurse who knew all the latest hygienic answers." Intrigued, she decided to experiment. She boarded out the sickliest newborns in the hopeless ward to a corps of gushing Italian mothers on the Lower East Side who had been trained in proper child care by the bureau's visiting nurses. "Off-hand it sounds like murder," Baker confesses. "Moving these poor little potential ghosts out of this ward where everything was light and sterile and spick and span, into tenement rooms on Hester and Orchard streets."

Once again the results were astonishing: The death rate of these vulnerable babies was cut in half. Baker had hit upon a truth that we now take for granted. At the time, medical opinion held that mothers should train their babies early to be independent by feeding them at regular intervals and ignoring their cries and babbles. Doing otherwise was thought to damage them psychologically and create neuroses. We now know the opposite is true. Emotionally sensitive and responsive human contact is essential for normal child development. Without such care, children may be physically stunted, mentally retarded, or even die.* Baker had no children of her own, but she saw clearly that though a baby "may still be unable to talk, walk or do anything but feed and cry and kick...he nevertheless needs that sense of being at home in a new world.... Even more than he needs butterfat and fresh air and clean diapers...he needs the personal equation to give him a reason for living."

That Baker's decisive work is so little known today is probably due to its great success: Much of what she taught us now seems self-evident. However, the neglect of her contributions may also be political. During the 1950s and '60s, America once again faced the challenge of integrating millions of disenfranchised citizens into its systems of public education, health, and social welfare, but this time those citizens were impoverished blacks, most of whom had been left behind by the public health revolution of the early twentieth century. They occupied, in demographer Samuel Preston's words, "a separate caste" in U.S. society. Their living conditions were much worse than those of whites, they had poorer access to whatever medical care was available, and black women with infants were much more likely to work outside the home—and for much longer hours and in much worse conditions than white women. This would have made it difficult for them to take advantage of the new health education and provide the kind of care their children needed.

Civil rights legislation and new programs like Medicare, Med-

---

*Karen Weintraub, "Structural Brain Changes Found in Romanian Orphanage Children," *CommonHealth*, July 23, 2012, available at http://commonhealth.wbur. org/2012/07/brain-changes-orphanage; R. A. Spitz, "Hospitalism: An Inquiry into the Genesis of Psychiatric Conditions in Early Childhood," *Psychoanalytic Study of the Child* 1 (1945): 53–74; and Wayne Dennis, *Children of the Crèche* (New York: Appleton-Century-Crofts, 1973).

icaid, and Head Start helped many people, both black and white, but they could not shield children from the steadily worsening poverty of the 1970s and '80s. In 1971, a group of Washington officials and their allies in the civil rights movement drafted the Comprehensive Child Care and Development Act, which would have created a nationwide system of high-quality day-care, preschool, and home-visiting programs that resembled the national system of child health programs envisioned by Baker and other reformers fifty years earlier. Most Americans supported the bill and it passed both houses of Congress with strong bipartisan support, but right-wing Republicans, using language similar to that used to quash the mother and baby care programs, pressured President Nixon to veto it.*

His adviser Pat Buchanan encouraged conservative journalists to write commentaries with headlines such as "Child Development Act—To Sovietize Our Youth," which Buchanan would then present to Nixon in his morning press digest, as if it represented mainstream conservative opinion.† Even though polls suggested most Americans supported the bill, large numbers of letters denouncing it—some even comparing it to the Hitler Youth programs—poured in to the White House. Edward Zigler, head of Nixon's Office of Child Development and one of the main architects of the bill, read through many of them. Most seemed to him to be form letters, and he suspected the campaign had been orchestrated by a small number of conservative opponents. Nevertheless, the president got the message, vetoed the bill, and the "Family Values" movement—devoted to challenging all federal programs for

---

*The Raising of America: Early Childhood and the Future of Our Nation (California Newsreel, 2013).
†Edward Zigler, The Hidden History of Head Start (Oxford University Press, 2010).

the poor—was born. Today, nearly every other industrialized nation on earth provides some form of guaranteed support to families with young children. That America still does not is considered by many to be a national disgrace.

After the veto, some experts continued to pursue the vision of comprehensive child care services. During the 1970s, David Olds, now a professor of pediatric psychiatry at the University of Colorado, was working in a Baltimore day-care center for preschoolers. Many of the children came from homes wracked by poverty, drug abuse, domestic violence, and other problems. Realizing that there was only so much the center could do to help them, he eventually went on to create the Nurse Family Partnership, a home-visiting program in which trained nurses taught poor mothers how to provide a safe, secure, stimulating environment for their children, and helped them envision a better future for themselves. Twenty years later, Olds found that the children of mothers who received the visits were not only healthier but were also less likely to have been abused or neglected and more likely to finish school, get jobs, and stay out of jail than a similar group of children whose mothers had not received the visits. Economists now estimate that every dollar invested in high quality home-visiting, day-care, and preschool programs results in $7 in savings on welfare payments, health-care costs, substance abuse treatment, and incarceration, plus higher tax revenues due to better-paying jobs.*

In the early 1930s, Baker toured Soviet Russia. Unlike the United States even now, the Soviets already had a comprehensive system of

---

*James J. Heckman and Dimitriy V. Masterov, "The Productivity Argument for Investing in Young Children," Working Paper 5, Invest in Kids Working Group (Committee for Economic Development, October 2004).

day-care centers and preschools. Maternal and child health care were free and pregnant women were given paid leave from their jobs. Baker was well aware of the purges, labor camps, deliberate mass starvation, and other horrors of the Soviet system, but the national dedication to the care of the young impressed her. Still, as she toured these programs, she noticed something odd. None of the children ever seemed to fight or cry, and she never saw children laughing, except on propaganda posters. "They just sat and looked at you like so many little Buddhas," she writes. Play activities were rigidly organized and even potty behavior seemed to be governed by Soviet methods of synchronized regulation.

Since its inception, the Soviet Union had been preparing for another world war, and Baker suspected there was a connection between this and the child-development programs. "You could not talk to any Intourist guide for ten minutes without hearing something about the Red Army and the impending war," she wrote, "and, from sickening experience, I knew it was no accident that, in 1934, the two groups of Russians who looked really well fed were the soldiers and the children."

In some respects, contemporary America is not all that different. It turns out there is one group of Americans that receives high-quality government-subsidized child-care services, including day care, preschool, home-visiting programs, and health care: the U.S. military. Unlike the Soviet version, these comprehensive programs aren't designed to create obedient little soldiers. Instead, they use a play-oriented approach to help bring out children's individual cognitive and social capabilities. This may help explain why military children score higher on reading and mathematics tests than public school children, and why the black/white achievement gap is much lower in military families than it is in the general population.*

---

*Michael Winerip, "Military Children Stay a Step Ahead of Public School Stu-

INTRODUCTION

Since the military child-care program was created in 1989, the government has repeatedly declined requests to fund an in-depth evaluation, perhaps because if the effects were known, all Americans would demand these programs for their children too.

Baker appears to have destroyed all her personal papers, so little is known about her life except what's in this memoir. After retiring from the Bureau of Child Hygiene, she lived in Princeton, New Jersey, with the novelist and Hollywood scriptwriter I.A.R. (Ida) Wylie, who was the author of more than a dozen romantic melodramas, including *Torch Song* with Joan Crawford and *Keeper of the Flame* with Spencer Tracy. The witty, detached, sometimes hilarious but always morally decent tone of *Fighting for Life* resembles Wylie's own memoir, *My Life with George*. Although the books tell totally different stories, some phrases, including "fighting for life," appear in both, and it's likely that Wylie ministered to Baker's prose. Their roommate was Louise Pearce, a Rockefeller University scientist who helped invent the cure for sleeping sickness and then traveled alone to the Belgian Congo in 1922 to test it. Around Princeton they were referred to as "the girls," but otherwise, gossip appears to have been restrained. They must have been wonderful to know. Read the first page of *Fighting for Life*, and you'll see.

—Helen Epstein

dents," *The New York Times*, December 12, 2011, available at http://www.nytimes.com/2011/12/12/education/military-children-outdo-public-school-students-on-naep-tests.html?pagewanted=all.

FIGHTING FOR LIFE

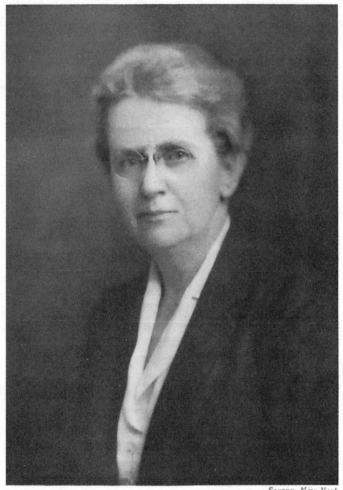

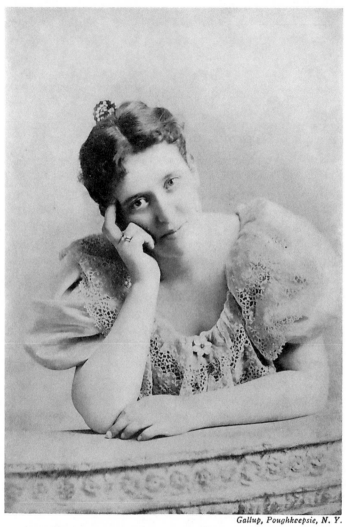

JUST BEFORE ENTERING MEDICAL COLLEGE, 1894

CHAPTER I

MY IMPULSE TO TRY TO DO THINGS ABOUT
hopeless situations appears to have cropped out first when
I was about six years old, and it should be pointed out that
the method I used was characteristically direct. I was all
dressed up for some great occasion—a beautiful white lacy
dress with a blue sash and light blue silk stockings and light
blue kid shoes—and inordinately vain about it. While
waiting for Mother to come down, I wandered out in front
of the house to sit on the horse block and admire myself
and hope that someone would come along and see me in all
my glory.

Presently a spectator did arrive—a little colored girl
about my size but thin and peaked and hungry looking,
wearing only a ragged old dress the color of ashes. I have
never seen such dumb envy in any human being's face before or since. Child that I was, I could not stand it; it
struck me right over the heart. I could not bear the idea
that I had so much and she had so little. So I got down off
the horse block and took off every stitch I had on, right
down to the blue shoes that were the joy of my infantile
heart and gave everything, underwear and all, to the little
black girl. I watched her as she scampered away, absolutely
choked with bliss. Then I walked back into the house, completely naked, wondering why I had done it and how to
explain my inexplicable conduct. Oddly enough both Father
and Mother seemed to understand pretty well what had

gone on in my mind. They were fine people, my father and mother.

I know that women of my generation who struck out on their own are supposed to have become rebellious because they felt cramped and suppressed and unhappy as children in an alien environment. It is a convenient formula and no doubt perfectly applicable in many cases. But it does not fit mine. I was reared in a thoroughly conventional tradition and took to it happily. I understood that after I left school I would go to Vassar, and then, I supposed, I would get married and raise a family and that would be that. Until events of the sort that are notoriously beyond one's control forced me to take bewildered thought for the morrow, I had no more purpose in life than a million other American girls being brought up just as I was in the eighties and nineties.

It would have taken a pretty demanding, not to say peevish, kind of child to fail to adjust to the family environment in which I was reared. We were reasonably well to do as wealth went in Poughkeepsie, so I had none of that precocious sense of responsibility which children often derive from straitened family incomes. Father was one of the most eminent lawyers in town; so eminent that, when I was making a speech in Poughkeepsie several years ago, I received a large basket of flowers with a card: "From the members of the Dutchess County Bar to the daughter of O. D. M. Baker." That was about thirty years after his death and it went straight to the heart of a daughter one of whose earliest resolves was to make it up to Father for having been born a girl. There is no particular point in emphasizing that ambition or its cause. Father was not one of those childish people who take disappointment out on children. But I did happen to arrive in the world as the

[2]

third daughter in a row and I heard family legends about Father's remarks when the nurse congratulated him on Daughter Number Three. Father always knew his own mind. He had known his own mind ever since he was a boy, when he ran away from a stepmother he disliked and educated himself into becoming a proverbially brilliant lawyer. The education was his first brilliant piece of work. He was one of those rare examples of self-educated people who really are educated.

He did things thoroughly. His professional education was sound and adequate. When he bought shoes, made to order in New York City, he ordered them seven pairs at a time, all exactly alike, and wore each pair only one day a week which, of course, was the best possible way to get maximum mileage out of each pair. When he went in for amateur carpentry for relaxation from the strain of business, he filled the attic with five times as many elaborate tools as the ordinary cabinetmaker uses, and became a first-class craftsman. He had been devoted to fishing all of his life. When he died, his fishing equipment included thirty-nine split bamboo rods, not to mention all kinds of odd tackle, and nearly thirteen thousand artificial flies all arranged around in cases in his library. By the time I could stand alone I was being taught to cast a line and every summer we spent a month or two at the Balsam Lake Club in the Catskill Mountains where we all fished in the Beaverkill Creek or in the quiet mountain lake which was part of the club's property. There were odd times of fishing in the Dutchess County lakes and streams and I can still drop a fly in an eddy with a subtlety that bodes ill for trout in the vicinity.

A sober, quiet man who never uttered an unnecessary word. His mother, who died when he was quite young, must have had romantic ambitions for him, because she named him: Orlando Daniel Mosher Baker. When he ran away from home, he came to Poughkeepsie from his nearby birthplace in Hyde Park, and was presently studying law in the office of the Honorable Homer A. Nelson. One day Mr. Nelson asked his young clerk to dinner to meet a young Vassar girl named Jenny Brown whose father, worried by the idea of having a daughter away from home at a new-fangled college, had asked his friend, Mr. Nelson, to look out for her. The bright young clerk and the pretty college girl liked each other on sight and the inevitable happened.

There were some fine and strange names in my family background, on my mother's side. My grandmother Brown was born in Boston. She was Arvilla Danforth, a direct descendant of the Samuel Danforth who was one of the committee to vote the money which made possible the founding of Harvard College. There was a curious trend in that branch of the Danforth family for they named their four daughters Arvilla, Permilla, Lucilla and Marilla. I knew only my grandmother, a fine woman of the old school, and my great-aunt Marilla who married Dr. Bleeker L. Hovey of Rochester, New York, and went with him as a nurse throughout the war between the states. As plain Jenny Brown, my mother inherited nothing of this richness of nomenclature; but she had a touch of the pioneer in her, a natural result of the same spirit which led her father, Merritt H. Brown who was born in Bennington, Vermont, to take his bride from Boston and trek out to the little settlement in Dansville, New York. There he and his wife brought up their family of seven children. My mother, who was the next to the youngest child, started out in the same spirit when she went to Poughkeepsie and, on the first day of the opening of Vassar College, enrolled herself as a student there. By pure chance, or perhaps by alphabetical arrangement, she appears on the record as the first, or one of the first, students to enter Matthew Vassar's new college for women. Fifty years after her enrollment, she was a guest of honor at the College's celebration of its half-century of progress and saw herself, in the college play, *Milestones*, as "Jenny Brown" portrayed in old-fashioned costume entering the college and talking to Matthew Vassar.

Our Poughkeepsie house was a fine sample of a kind of architecture which has left an ineffaceable mark on Hudson River towns: three stories, gray slate mansard roof, veranda across the front, patch of front lawn and a stretch of back lawn running through to the next street, decorated with trees and a children's play house. All it lacked to be perfect was a set of lightning rods. Evidently Father was one of the few citizens of Poughkeepsie sufficiently strong minded to resist the blandishments of the ever-present lightning-rod salesman. My father and mother went to live in this house when they were first married and we four children were all born there. My oldest sister, Arvilla, died in infancy; my next older sister, Mary, lived until about twelve years ago; my brother, Robert Nelson Millerd Baker, died when he was thirteen; and now I am the only one left of that vigorous and very happy family.

There was plenty of room in our house and we made the most of it. Only on rare occasions were we without guests. It seemed to me that there were always people coming or going or staying. Innumerable friends made it a stopping place. There were my numerous cousins from Amherst College who always came for the holidays and many of the students from the thriving Riverside Military School in town which had a great reputation as an educational institution in those days and drew boys from all over the United States. There were *always* relays of Vassar students who would come for the week ends and bring with them any girls who they thought looked homesick. Dr. Kendrick, who was then the President of Vassar, used to call it "The Vassar Annex," but it was more than that. I belonged to a hospitable family.

There was little to Vassar College at that time but the old main building, a gymnasium and the astronomical observatory which naturally followed from the fact that Maria Mitchell, the great woman astronomer, was a member of the faculty. It was strict, too, much stricter than the present-day girls' boarding school. The girls were not allowed even to come into Poughkeepsie without a teacher as an escort, though that seemed to be waived when they came to see us. We knew all about it and were as much at home with the personnel of the institution as if they had been our cousins. Commencement time, Founders Day, and "Phil" would mean as much company and jollification as Christmas and always rated with circus day in my juvenile calendar.

It took something big to be a great occasion too, for people lived gaily in that era. I do not know what charts of the business cycle have to say about it, but as I look back, it seems to me to have been an ample, affluent time. I think the gay nineties deserved their name; certainly the earlier part of that decade was a joyous time and even before that we were gay enough; even the children were.

There was always something going on, some simple, cheerful, comradely occasion among people who all knew and liked each other. We took full advantage of being on the Hudson River and one of my major accolades of that time was when the Poughkeepsie paper said that I pulled "one of the best oars among the girls in town." There were the clam bakes which were held a few miles up the river, the kind of clam bakes that are rare today. Starting with a stone-lined pit in the ground which in preparation was heated to a white heat, the ashes were cleaned away and then successive layers of bluefish, chicken, green corn and dozens of clams were covered over to bake into a delectable meal fit for the gods. There were picnics and boating parties in plenty and, when the first college boat race of the big Poughkeepsie rowing regatta was instituted, we knew everyone connected with the management and I saw this first race from the judges' launch, which has spoiled me ever since for anything so distantly dull as an observation train along the bank of the river. In the winter our life became even more exciting with ice-skating and ice-boating on the frozen Hudson. It is an easy cliché to say that the seasons have changed, but our winters then were long and cold and the river was solidly frozen over for weeks.

Skating kept you warm in your own right, but you came back from an icy cruise at lightning speed on an ice-boat almost as frozen as the Hudson. Ice-yachting was rare sport when one could lie out at full length in the tiny cockpit and fly along, often on one runner, racing with the crack trains along the bank and often making a speed of sixty miles an hour. But you wanted it to be cold, knife-blade cold in the moonlight with a big fire glowing on the bank to come back to just when you thought your face and feet would never be able to thaw out again. There was bob-sledding on the long hills in town when ten or twelve of us would pile ourselves on the long sled and start off on what seemed to us a perilous trip. We always found some friendly horses and driver who would pull us up the hill

[7]

again to repeat the performance. Sometimes in the evening and effectively chaperoned, a dozen or fifteen youngsters would pile into a long, four-horse sled, packed with straw, and drive out into the country to a special farmhouse where huge bowls of oyster stew would be waiting when the sled's runners creaked in the yard. On the way home we sang like frogs in the spring, sang "My Bonnie Lies Over the Ocean" and "Seeing Nellie Home" and "Clementine" and "After the Ball Is Over" and that song about a bicycle built for two.

Whether in town or country things were simply and generously managed in my world. The whole family were always going on visits into the country, old-fashioned, pre-commuter Dutchess County country, perhaps to a relative's house, perhaps to that of a prosperous farmer who was a client of Father's. The home was always a lovely old place and completely innocent of heating in the bedrooms. The family were usually realists and slept in woolen sheets all winter. But, winter or not, we city folks, who also were guests of honor, had beautiful home-woven linen sheets on our beds and froze to death in consequence. It was worth it, however, in view of the breakfast you would get after arising and dressing with your breath smoking in front of you. You breakfasted in the comfortable great kitchen, cheek by jowl with the huge Dutch oven where the bread was baked and all the other cooking done over the roaring fire; breakfasted on huge bowls of oatmeal, ham and eggs, sausages, pork chops, steak, fried potatoes, stacks of hot biscuits and mounds of griddle cakes. Those breakfasts are among my most vivid childhood memories and I cannot today pass the old Perkins place on the South Road without a nostalgic feeling for the wholly lovely week ends I have spent there. There's no denying it, children are greedy little things and to make an impression on their stomachs is the surest way to be remembered.

At appropriate seasons, in town, there were candy-pulls, more formal luncheons, dances galore with the fast and swooping waltzes, the polka and the redowa, for dancing was active exercise in those days. We had many cotillions then with gay favors, cotillions which we began in our dancing-school days and I kept up until I left home. There were the gay balls which followed the annual visits of the Yale or Harvard or Amherst College Glee Club to our town. One of my loveliest remembrances is of the year when I was lame and the entire Amherst Glee Club came up to our house in the afternoon and gave me, as sole audience, their entire program of the evening's concert to which I couldn't go. In the summer, in later years, there was tennis; I became a fairly acceptable player and won many tournaments in the Hudson River towns. I do not mean that all this happened when I was a child. It is all mixed up in my memory for, until I was seventeen, the world was a unit with no gaps or turning points. It all seems very hectic and gay as I look back upon it.

Of course I can find a few special characteristics creeping out, if I look for them. Trying to make it up to Father for being a girl, which went right on even after the next arrival delighted the household by being a boy, did turn me into a tomboy type in the early days. I was an enthusiastic baseball player and trout-fisher and still like both of these amusements fifty years later. My pet reading was neither Elsie Dinsmore nor fairy stories, but the classic stories of Horatio Alger, Jr., and *Toby Tyler, or Ten Weeks with a Circus* as it appeared in that lovable old magazine, *Harper's Young People*. The circus was very important in my life. The night before the circus came to town, my brother and I always went to bed with strings tied to our toes and dangling out of the windows. Our confederate was the local Poughkeepsie bad boy, whom we were forbidden to know and whom, in consequence, we cultivated on every possible occasion. As soon as the circus arrived, he ran to our house and jerked the strings. We got up, dressed and crept out and went down to the circus lot where they were unloading elephants and erecting tents with shouting and heaving on ropes and hammering in stakes with smashing sledge hammers, all in the weird, savage light of kerosene flares. Then, so dazzled and excited we felt a little sick, back we stole just as it was getting light, undressed and got back into bed in time to be summoned from below: "Children! Get up at once or you will be late for school!" Lots of Poughkeepsie youngsters would be unaccountably drowsy in school on circus day, but they were all boys except me. And for weeks after the circus left my brother and I did nothing but play at being "Mademoiselle Jeannette and Monsieur Ajax, the World's Most Graceful and Daring Aerial Artistes" on the trapeze in our play-house.

My brother and I also collaborated in the manufacture and use of tick-tacks, particularly for the stirring up of two rather timid middle-aged ladies who lived next door. Our style of tick-tack consisted of a long cord, a small pebble and a pin. You put the pin in the window sash so the pebble dangled against the pane and then stood far off and gently twitched the other end of the cord, which made the pebble rap insistently on the glass—tap-tap-tap . . . tap-tap-tap . . . until the frightened ladies roused up, the gas was lighted, and quavering voices were heard: "Who's there?" As soon as there was any risk of detection, you gave a hearty tug on the cord, which pulled out the pin and removed all traces of the crime. Occasionally we moved farther afield and stirred up other mystified households.

Tick-tacks were not, however, part of our Hallowe'en program. Hallowe'en was just a matter of parties where you bobbed for apples and walked backward down the cellar-stairs looking into a mirror for a possible glimpse of your future husband—for girls anyway. The boys were apparently more active, since the horse-block, which then stood in front of every house with the householder's name carved on it like a tombstone, was usually found next morning overturned into the gutter and a good many gates would be temporarily missing. I always had the impression that part of Father's and Mother's idea in giving us Hallowe'en parties was to keep us in the house and out of mischief. We did not wear funny costumes on Hallowe'en, however. That was the custom at Thanksgiving when we dressed ourselves in Mother's clothes and went to call on our neighbors. Youngsters had little to do with New Year's except to stay at home in their best clothes and make raids on the sandwiches and cakes which surrounded the open-house punch bowl. Everyone kept open house on New Year's Day; the ladies stayed at home and "received" and the gentlemen paid calls to all the ladies they knew. A fine old-fashioned custom that called for a steady head. By the time a widely acquainted bachelor had paid thirty or forty calls and drunk a cup of punch to a happy New Year for the household at every port of call, he was likely to be precariously merry and need a good deal of expert steering. I will say for the credit of our visitors, however, that relatively few of them ever disgraced the dignity of the silk hat and Prince Albert coat which was the required uniform for the occasion.

There are all sorts of memories which come back to me of those carefree days. Our domestic circle had an unusual stability during all my years at home. It is a strange commentary upon the changing servant problem of today when I remember that Bridget, the cook, Mary, the maid, Mrs. Uniack, the laundress, and Frances, our colored nurse of blessed memory, were with us always. Frances was our other mother and my love for and sympathy with and understanding of the colored race date back to her and all she meant to us children. There was Smith's candy store on Market Street. It is still there but without the presence of William and Andrew Smith with their delectable beards and their great sense of fine citizenship. They may be known now as "Trade" and "Mark," but to me they were great men and their generosity to the town remains as their monument. There was the old barn on Church Street where they were beginning to manufacture the cough drops which were to make them famous, then little known and made in a primitive way. We children used to go in to watch the black drops coming slowly out on narrow sheets of tin and always went away with our pockets full. There were the afternoons much later when Cornelia Kinkead and I used to visit each other and sit for long hours, each immersed in a book and rarely speaking to the other. There was our mandolin and guitar club ably led by Anna Haight, who was a distinguished musician and who made us able to give rather charming little musical afternoons. There were "progressive" card parties and the old friendships of kindred souls. All muddled memories, stretching over the years of childhood and youth, and all precious as a reminder of a life in a small town for a young girl in the eighties and nineties. Traditional small-town stuff, it may be, but I doubt if the world offers anything better today. It was a good world that I lived in.

I was thoroughly trained in the business of being a

woman. My sister Mary and I went through rigorous education in cooking and sewing; no superficial bowing acquaintance with cook-stove and sewing-machine, but real work.
That was a hold-over from my mother's education and almost necessary when the corner grocery had little but
staples on its shelves and the ready-made dress had not yet
developed into a major industry. Twice a year the dress-
maker came to the house and stayed six weeks at a time
making summer or winter outfits for Mother, my sister
and myself, and part of her job was to make seamstresses
of Mary and me. I could make my own clothes now, if I
wanted to. Modern clothes would be all too simple. I was
trained when a dress was a dress, a creation of complicated
architecture, stiffened with whalebone, gored, ruffled, covered with darts and loops and fancy stitching.

Cooking was the same way. Every year we put up a
year's supply of jams and jellies and preserves, and it was
a family tradition that no daughter of the house could
qualify as on the way to growing up until she could cook
a dinner that would pass muster with Father. And he was
a severe judge. Father liked his food and had high standards in culinary matters, so I know I am a good cook. I do
not cook and I do not like to cook and I have not done it
for many years, but I feel quite confident that I could walk
out into my own kitchen tomorrow and bake bread that
would be a credit to our old Bridget. And I can still manage a coal range, which is becoming a lost art among town-
bred young women.

Summers were mostly spent at my grandmother's in
Dansville, the loveliest of little towns nestling at the head
of the Genesee Valley in New York State. Our house in
Poughkeepsie was sizable, but it was cramped in comparison to Grandmother's white-pillared place on Elizabeth

[15]

Street. There was always plenty of room even though my grandmother had seven children and six of them married and had families and they all sent all of the grandchildren to her in the summer. And plenty of welcome too: I cannot understand how either the house or Grandmother's patience held together, but it was a sturdy old building and she was the kindliest and least irritable of old ladies and unmistakably loved having us there.

Every year I revelled in Dansville and the effects will never wear off. Just last year, in the *Saturday Evening Post*, I read a story by Hugh MacNair Kahler about a small town which gave me a strangely reminiscent feeling; the background was slight but I knew that place. We live now in the Kahler home in Princeton, and the next time I saw my landlord I asked him if he had any particular place in mind when he wrote that story. "Why yes," he said, "but you have probably never been there; very few people have. It's a little town in upstate New York called Dansville." Whereupon it developed that he had been raised in the place and was one of the MacNair grandchildren with whom we Brown grandchildren had played—and presumably fought—summer after summer.

I have an idea that he has obtained a great deal of material for his stories from Dansville. If it were not for the limitations of this book and the need of getting on to my main purpose in life, I could recite all sorts of minor Dansville sagas, for it is one of those small towns that breed stories. It has a way of staying with you and if you turned me loose today blindfolded in Dansville I should know where I was.

The old town has changed a great deal in these forty-odd years. The bloomer-clad, skull-capped, Dutch-cut-haired ladies from old Dr. Jackson's health resort up on

[14]

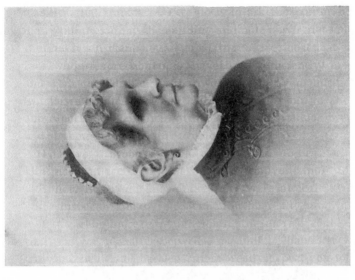

MERRITT HOLMES BROWN
My maternal grandfather

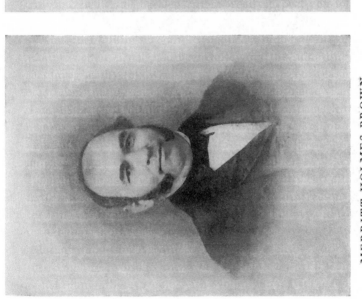

ARVILLA DANFORTH BROWN
My maternal grandmother

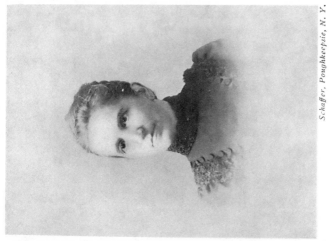

Schaffer, Poughkeepsie, N. Y.

JENNY HARWOOD BAKER

My mother

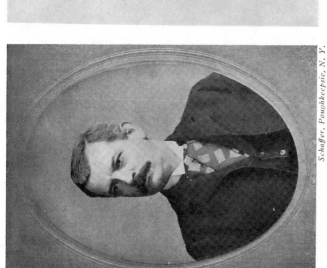

Schaffer, Poughkeepsie, N. Y.

O. D. M. BAKER

My father

the hill are no longer there, and that is a great loss. Dr. Jackson was a fine-looking, white-bearded and jolly old gentleman who had picturesque ideas about health and carried them out to the ultimate degree in this establishment. He frowned on meat, so meat was barred. He believed heartily in eating cereals and fruit, so they were ever present. He made, and had his patients eat, what I believe was the first prepared breakfast food: a really delicious concoction called "granula." I have often been there for supper. The patients sat at long tables in the dining room, between which ran a narrow-gauge railroad track. The huge bell on top of the building clanged once and a handcar heaped with hard graham biscuit, the inevitable "granula," and apple sauce appeared out of the sliding doors at the end of the room. That was supper, washed down with copious glassfuls of water. Dr. Jackson believed even more heartily in the curative properties of a spring up on the hillside above the building. It was called the All-Healing Spring and was just good spring water.

Long ago, Dr. Amelia Bloomer had convinced Dr. Jackson that skirts were a menace to health, so all of his women patients had to wear the semi-Turkish trousers named after their inventor. There also seemed something lethal about long hair, although I never understood just what it was, which made it necessary for the same long-suffering ladies to have their hair cut short in a Dutch bob and wear little skull caps on their heads. They looked very strange and unworldly to this small child. Many of them were apparently sane when observed by an inquisitive little girl down the hill on Dansville's main street. Maybe the doctor's regimen did do them some good; at least he never lacked for patients.

When the doctor died—at eighty-five, a good testimonial for his system of living—his son and daughter-in-law, Drs. James and Kate Jackson, inherited the place and started letting down some of the bars. While they were thinking about this, the Sanitarium burned down. The excitement of this great event prostrated Dansville for days. I was there, at my grandmother's, at that time. I remember a great glare in the sky and the knock on my grandmother's door. When answered, it proved to herald a patient from the Sanitarium who, having been unable to walk for years, had been startled by the cry of fire into getting out of bed, throwing her case of jewels out of the window, deliberately picking up the bowl and pitcher from her washstand and walking in her nightgown all the way down the hill. The bowl and pitcher were just one of those queer things people do in emergencies. I can thus vouch for at least one cure effected in the Jackson Sanitarium. They never did find the jewels.

The Sanitarium was rebuilt in red brick, started up on a much more liberal basis by the younger Dr. Jackson, and prospered exceedingly. The bloomers, the hair-cuts and the skull-caps were discarded and in my medical days I worked there for two summers as a laboratory technician, gaining invaluable practical experience in making analyses and having a very pleasant time. William Dean Howells was there as a patient one summer and having tea with him in the afternoon was a thrilling episode in my young life. The place caught a celebrity like that quite often. Possibly the one that meant the most to me was Louisa M. Alcott. I wish I could remember more about her. She seemed to be just a very gentle and very tired old lady. She was my heroine of all the world at that time, and a proper choice if I was going to strike out on my own in the world, though nothing could have been farther from my thoughts then. For Louisa M. Alcott was, to me, the unattainable ideal of a great woman. *Little Women* and *Little Men* were favorite reading everywhere I turned among girls of my own age and "Jo" in *Little Women* has always been my favorite character in all fiction. I feel a glow of happiness, even today, when I find that these books are still read and loved. And so, to have met Louisa M. Alcott and to have known her, even so slightly, remains one of my precious memories.

The old doctor's grandson, also a doctor, inherited the Sanitarium in his turn and liberalized it still more. It is still there; but it was sold recently to Bernarr Macfadden for a health resort, to be run according to his theories. In other words, it has completed the cycle and come back to where it started from: three generations from cracked wheat to cracked wheat. I hope Mr. Macfadden's patients are as picturesque as old Dr. Jackson's were, but I doubt it. Anyway, I congratulate Mr. Macfadden upon his inheritance of a fine tradition.

I know that New York City has lost a great deal of its dash and glamour since the time when the whole family used to go on board the *Mary Powell*, the queen of the old Hudson River boats, and come to the city for a day of shopping and the theater. Without sounding like a professional admirer of the good old days, I do want to put myself on record to the effect that, whatever its numerous advantages, the modern world does not know how to live as comfortably as did the world of the nineties. There are no more hotels like the old Fifth Avenue Hotel, where we always stayed, with its palatial, roomy, black-tiled lobby and its mammoth bedrooms full of carved black walnut furniture (the huge, comfortable beds cured countless cases of insomnia) and those enormous bills of fare in the restaurant, where you ate three meals a day—getting room, breakfast, lunch and dinner for five dollars per person. It would have taken half an hour merely to read the breakfast menu through, so you stopped somewhere down among the tenderloin steaks and baked potatoes and ordered anything you thought of, secure in the well-justified confidence that it would be forthcoming.

I have a nostalgic feeling for the theater in those days too. After the lapse of years it is impossible for me to get all of the actors into their proper places. (There are plenty of books that will tell you all that, but I know that my education was singularly rich in all the stage could give.) Names come tumbling over themselves in my mind; different years, but all in my younger life. The cozy little Lyceum Theater on the corner of Twenty-third Street and Fourth Avenue where the seats all folded back so that the whole theater became a sea of aisles. The grand, and new, Empire Theater way uptown at Fortieth Street and Broadway. Both with magnificent stock companies where each player was a star. Weber and Fields Music Hall and the old Tony Pastor place on Fourteenth Street. I saw Sarah Bernhardt and heard Adelina Patti sing on the last of her many "farewell tours." There were Henry Irving and Ellen Terry, and I saw Maude Adams and Ethel Barrymore make their debuts. The music halls gave their quota: Lottie Collins, whose Ta-Ra-Ra-Boom-De-Ay set all the town singing; Weber and Fields, Blanche Ring, Vesta Tilley, Cecilia Loftus, Della Fox, Willie Collier, Albert Chevalier, Dan Daly, Lillian Russell, Nat Goodwin and DeWolf Hopper. I know I have left many out of this long-ago list but it was a rich galaxy and I am glad to have lived so long if only to have seen and heard them all.

The stores we patronized were all quite handy to the

old horse-drawn streetcar that brought us over from the dock where the *Mary Powell* landed because few if any stores had then crept above Twenty-third Street. The famous Delmonico's, just above Madison Square, was almost as far north as we ever went on these trips. Many of the names will sound familiar to modern ears, but the locations are changed now. Arnold Constable's and Lord & Taylor's were on Broadway near Seventeenth Street; Altman's at Sixth Avenue and Eighteenth Street right on the Elevated, where no smart store would dream of being now; Mc-Creery's on Broadway below Twenty-third Street and Macy's still at the corner of Fourteenth Street and Sixth Avenue. Three large department stores of those days are but blessed memories: Simpson, Crawford & Simpson, O'Neill's, and the famous "Meet me at the Fountain" emporium of Siegel-Cooper. By lunch time we probably got down as far as the old St. Denis Hotel, opposite Grace Church, and a lunch there was something to dream about, even better than the good French cooking they served you at the sit-up counter at Purcell's across the street.

Today's youngsters evidently think that a girl's life in the nineties must have been unendurably confining, to match those elaborate whalebone-stiffened clothes she wore. But it seems to me that there is not much that today offers which would compensate for the gay and free days of my youth. There were a great many more "don'ts" to observe then than there are now. But there were also plenty of occasions when the "don'ts" grew transparent and started you to wondering what was underneath. There was, for instance, my Aunt Abby who gave me my first acquaintance with skepticism and non-conformity. I could not begin to explain Aunt Abby but I know she was an invaluable part of my education.

She was my father's Aunt, one of a large family of old-fashioned Quakers, whose use of plain language always made ordinary English words sound silvery and beautiful. When I first remember her, she was nearly a hundred years old, a tiny old lady in severe Quaker gray with a white 'kerchief about her neck and her bonnet strings tied underneath her chin in a great gray bow. Quakers have a way of being different without anyone's minding; perhaps I had more of that quality in me than anyone realized. I know that there were two diverse elements in me struggling for expression: the gay, social and ambitious expression of my mother's personality and the quiet, taciturn and withdrawn calmness of my father's Quaker upbringing. . . . But to come back to my Aunt Abby. Her particular crotchet was turning day into night, just like Marcel Proust, of all people. She got up and had her breakfast at midnight, ate her dinner when the sun was coming up over the horizon, had her supper at eleven A.M. and then went to bed again at noon. Her son, with whom she lived on a big farm a few miles outside of Poughkeepsie, would never have dreamed of expostulating with her about her strange habits and she lived in one wing of the big house with her own maid to look after her.

So, if you wanted to see my great-aunt Abby, you had to get up at the crack of dawn in order to finish the long carriage ride out from town before she went to bed. We children were always eager to go for reasons of our own: we knew Aunt Abby's diabolical and thoroughly enticing secret, and Father and Mother did not. As soon as we arrived, Mother and Uncle James went off about their own concerns and left us children to Aunt Abby's ministrations. Then the thrilling performance began. Aunt Abby would settle her little self on the big old mahogany-and-haircloth sofa with the sampler on the wall over her head, her feet propped on a mahogany footstool embroidered with a gay parrot, range us in front of her on a haircloth footstool apiece, and call for her Bible. It was a colossal volume which practically smothered her when it was opened across her lap. The remarkable old lady never wore glasses and with her keen eyesight she would read us a Bible story, the most incredible she could find: it might be Jonah and the whale, or the three Israelites in the fiery furnace, or perhaps Daniel in the lions' den. It must have made a very pretty picture like an old steel engraving out of a child's book: the old lady, so long past the allotted three score years and ten, reading the Scripture to three curly-headed youngsters. She always read the story with much earnestness and we hung on each word. Then, closing the book, she would look up at us benignly and say:

"Now, children, that is a very silly story. I am an old, old lady and I want all of you to remember what I am saying. It is a silly story and there is not a word of truth in it. Don't ever let anyone tell you that stories like that are true. . . . Jane! Cookies!" Then we ate the cookies and enjoyed them almost as much as this secret display of thrilling skepticism. When Mother returned, she always heard only that Aunt Abby had been reading us Bible stories. We all continued regularly to go to Sunday school without rebellion, but it was hardly possible for us to take much stock in Jonah and the whale from that time on. It would probably be hard to exaggerate the influence that sort of experience may have on a child, learning so early that it is possible to question the unquestionable. We were thoroughly impressed but, although Aunt Abby never asked us not to, we never told anyone of these shocking adventures. When she died at the age of one hundred and six, we chil-

dren were the only ones who knew her secret. Everyone
else assumed that she died as she had apparently lived, an
ardent and absolutely believing Quaker. That was so long
ago that it can do no harm to tell about it now. And I am
not so sure, as I look back on this, of its effect on each of
us. My sister, Mary, became a religious devotee and her
complete interest in life was the so-called "High Church"
branch of the Protestant Episcopal Church. Perhaps my
mind was fertile soil for that seed: I know it was the beginning of my desire to question the right and wrong of all
accepted doctrines.

This all sounds as though life, for me, was a round of
good times and active gaieties. Life in my family with so
energetic a mother had to be that but there was no lack of
formal education. I was extremely fond of the school to
which I was sent. My attendance there covered all of my
school life except for one year when, for some inexplicable
reason, I was sent to another private school which carried
out its educational regime under the accepted plan. But I
was not altogether happy or contented there, and the following year saw me back in my old environment to stay
until my college years. It was a highly unusual school, of a
type practically unheard of fifty years ago, although some
of its peculiarities have much in common with the most advanced of modern educational methods. The school was the
private effort of the Misses Thomas, two extremely large
ladies who much resembled the late Elisabeth Marbury, in a
lovely, peaceful old house on Academy Street, full of ex-
quisite old furniture and a sense of overwhelming calm
which impressed the most rambunctious little girl the moment she entered. Miss Sarah conducted the teaching and
Miss "Lib" the housekeeping, for there were six or seven
boarders among the thirty-odd pupils. They were both im-

pressive people. Miss Sarah was stern and dignified but "Miss Lib" was known through all Dutchess County for her bubbling sense of humor and her ready wit. Once, for instance, when we were driving with her out into the country, we were being badly bothered by a buggy ahead which was smothering us with dust. Presently someone saw that the driver in the buggy ahead was the local undertaker, which made the situation about as dismal as possible. "Oh, I don't know," said Miss Lib, "I'd rather take his dust than have him take mine." One can still hear stories about Miss Lib, in Poughkeepsie.

So far as the academic side went, the school itself was strangely modern in its plan of study. There were no graded classes, no marks or reports, no examinations, not even any commencement exercises. When Miss Sarah was satisfied that you knew enough mathematics, Latin, French, English, or the elementary sciences, she told you so and all of the women's colleges of that time took her certificate of a student's preparation as sufficient for entrance requirements without a shadow of question. The classes were small and rather informal affairs with only three or four girls in each group, usually held around a table in some upstairs room. You progressed strictly according to your ability to master that particular course. If you had a special piece of work to do, you took your own time to master it, without urging. The teachers were nearly all college-bred women and the instruction was fine and thorough. Discipline was hardly needed, so beautifully did this pair of fine, shrewd women manage their charges. The most severe punishment meted out was having to stay in school after hours and learn twenty or thirty lines of some famous poem before going home. That took a good deal of time, theoretically, but practically we soon learned what

[23]

the poems would be—it was always the same one until we could recite it all. So we would learn the poem ahead of time, take half an hour or so during our punishment after school to make it seem plausible and then go free. For years and years after I left home I could still recite *Thanatopsis*, *The Lay of the Last Minstrel*, and parts of *The Idylls of the King*.

I have no idea where the Misses Thomas evolved their plan of conducting a school along these latitudinarian lines, any more than I can conceive how they managed to run it so successfully and smoothly that way. Naturally their curious ideas struck many residents of Poughkeepsie as too queer to be safe and there was a large body of substantial citizenry who insisted upon sending their daughters to the town's other and more conventional schools. But many of what I believe to have been the more progressive people, Father among them, were heartily in favor of it and I am very glad that his mind was tuned to that decision. It was splendid preparation for a child who would presently have to study on her own. By the time I was sixteen I was prepared to enter any women's college in the country and in Latin and mathematics could have been eligible for entrance to the Sophomore year.

There had never been any question about my entering Vassar, which was already as familiar to me as my own face in the mirror. But then things began to happen with devastating swiftness. That was just my private calamity out of a series of calamities which went far toward shattering our family and jarred me out of the life I was apparently destined to lead.

When I was sixteen my brother died suddenly. He was only thirteen years old but a fine and promising lad and the one boy in a family of girls. Three months later Father died of typhoid. In those days typhoid was the scourge of

Poughkeepsie and no wonder, since the town water supply was drawn from the Hudson just below the outlet of the sewer from the large Asylum for the Insane above the town. The epidemic of typhoid that winter had one good effect: it resulted in the installation of the first American filtration plant for a town's water supply. Father's typhoid was serious enough, but we all knew it was rather a lack of will to live that killed him. My brother's death had taken all the zest for life from him. We were an understanding trio—my father, my brother, and myself—and when they died so close together there seemed very little left to live for.

Perhaps it was just as well that financial troubles appeared so soon after Father's funeral to make us all think of something else. We had always had a comfortable home and enough money, and Father had saved too. But when the estate came to be settled, a recent series of losses and bad investments told the inevitable story of practically nothing left. It was immediately evident that somebody would have to get ready to earn a living for all three of us—my mother, my sister, who had always been delicate and a semi-invalid, and myself. I considered myself elected. It was a hard struggle to give up Vassar but there was not enough money left to pay for that and for any additional preparation for a professional life. I had long talks with Dr. Taylor who was then President of Vassar, and with Professor Leach who was determined that I should follow my original plan. A scholarship was ready for me but time loomed large when I thought of nine or ten years of study. I made my own decision, after months of agonizing debate, and in the end it was decided that Mother and Mary should live at home and I should take five thousand of the few precious dollars remaining, go to New York and study to be a doctor.

CHAPTER II

I WISH I COULD REMEMBER WHAT MADE ME choose medicine as a way of earning my living—for that is the conscious commercial attitude I had toward it at that time. I expect that even then I did not know my motive very clearly. Many years afterward, a newspaper reporter interviewed me for hours in an effort to get a story which would give some definite starting point to my career. He did not do so badly after all, for the completed article when published filled three columns of newspaper space. His conclusion was that an injury to my knee, which kept me on crutches for over two years, had developed in me a tremendous respect for the profession of medicine and a not-to-be-denied yearning for a medical education. To be exact he wrote: "If little Josephine Baker had not hurt her knee, 90,000 babies now alive would have died." I have the utmost respect for the Fourth Estate and in my years of Health Department work learned to know intimately many of those splendid fellows—of both sexes—and I know what "copy" means to a reporter. But I have a profound conviction that he was wrong. I did have a deep affection for the doctors who took care of me during that time. They were father and son, "old" Dr. Lewis Sayre and his son Dr. Lewis H. Sayre. The old doctor was New York's most celebrated orthopedist. He was the stiffest, most fiercely starched, the sternest and most likable martinet who ever practiced medicine. His older son was a gentle edition of his father. With the third son, Dr. Reginald Sayre, they formed an unforgettable trio in the best of the old medical tradition. But no one could have been more acid or more profoundly skeptical of women doctors than old Dr. Sayre was. When I once diffidently mentioned to him that I was thinking of studying medicine, the atmosphere was sulphuric with his comments. He ruthlessly discouraged me as did our own family physician Dr. John Kinkead. But later Dr. Kinkead, for whom I had a great admiration and affection, was a loyal, devoted friend who helped me over many bad places.

It was strange. I had known only one woman doctor at all well—Dr. Kate Jackson. I had barely heard that there were such people but was quite aware that the world did not wholly approve of them. I was to be in no sense a pioneer in the study and practice of medicine. But in my sheltered life medical women were such rare and unusual creatures that they could hardly be said to exist at all. There was no medical tradition on either side of my family. There were lawyers but no doctors. And both sides of the family were aghast at the idea of my spending so much money in such an unconventional way. It was an unheard of, a harebrained and unwomanly scheme. At first my mother too was rather overwhelmed at the idea, but she trusted me and she made a gallant surrender. "If you really think you should, Jo," she said, "go ahead. I'll try not to fret too much about it." Besides she had been through this sort of perplexity herself; it had taken a good deal of courage and determination to uproot oneself from a little town and experiment with a newly-founded women's college in 1861.

My only explanation of the mental process that led me to my decision is that the study of medicine did occur to me, rather casually, from my long association with the Doctors Sayre, and that later, when I encountered only argument and disapproval, my native stubbornness made me decide to study medicine at all costs and in spite of everyone. That is, after all, hardly a rational way to choose one's life work and yet, in a curious way, it seems to hold the secret of whatever success may come to one in later life. I am thoroughly convinced that obstacles to be overcome and disapproval to be lived down are strong motive forces. Years afterward, when I came into intimate contact with what has been called "the submerged tenth," I knew that this was true. The children of the rich and well-to-do with the way made easy for them have a hard and difficult road to travel; the children of the poor and underprivileged, battling against disabilities all their young lives, not only have a great incentive but are so used to hardships and discouragements that the future way may seem almost unbelievably easy. Everyone can see innumerable examples of the handicap of wealth and the stimulus of poverty. In my case the need of some such future outlet was imperative. My choice of medicine as a career turned out rather better than I deserved, for I was to learn that this profession demands not only stubbornness but a devotion so wholehearted that it amounts to absolute consecration.

For a great many years while I was with the New York City Health Department, there used to come into my office each spring a long line of young men and women each with the same question to ask: "Do you advise me to study medicine? I want to do something with my life and medicine seems a good career. I can't make up my mind about it and the preparation seems long and difficult. So I thought I would ask your advice about it." There is just one answer to that question and there never can be more than one answer. It is a final and emphatic "NO." There is something about the practice, and the study, of medicine that takes all of one's devotion, all of one's interest and, in most instances, all of one's life. I used to tell these doubtful young people just that. And the advice is as true today as it always has been. "If," I would say, "you are prepared to study medicine and determined to do it against all the advice of your friends and your family, if you are ready to go through with it even to the point of being disinherited, and if your decision is so definitely made that there can be no other course for you, then you wouldn't come to me with this question. The very fact that you are asking me to decide for you shows me that medicine is not for you nor you for medicine. You may study and become an average doctor but medicine, like the ministry, is a jealous mistress. Determination, courage, and a love of your fellow-man are its keynotes and nothing less will answer."

In the beginning I was one of these weak sisters. It took about six weeks of unaccustomed and unpleasant work for me to be transformed to the place where I could honestly say to myself: "This is the one thing of all others that I will and must do." I have never regretted it. Long hours of work both day and night, discouragement and rebuffs all seemed just part of a natural life and if it has been a difficult road to travel it has also been a deeply satisfying one.

When I began my bashful and inefficient inquiries as to the way of getting a medical education my ignorance was colossal. Finally some courageous good angel—I wish I could remember who it was—told me that there was a women's medical college in New York attached to the

New York Infirmary for Women and Children. That was
little enough to go on but it spurred me into going down
to New York and timidly assailing the place. It was a
pleasant building, on the corner of Stuyvesant Square at
East Fifteenth Street, and, when I summoned up my courage to go in and ask questions, they treated me very well.
It was a brisk, and yet a serious institution. I liked it and
found with great relief that the people in charge—all
women too—seemed to consider the study of medicine a
reasonable career for a girl. But they made it clear that I
should have to earn my opportunity. The certificate from
Miss Thomas which would enable me to enter Vassar College was of no value here. This college required a certificate from the State Board of Regents covering a series of
subjects which included elementary chemistry and biology.
In order to get the required counts, I should have to pass
examinations in all of the elementary subjects that belonged to my earliest school days.

So back home I went and for the next year I studied
continuously and renewed my acquaintance with arithmetic, geography and even spelling (which continues to be
one of my weakest points). I was near enough to studies
like Latin, French and the higher mathematics to have
them cause me no difficulty. But the States bounding the
Mississippi River and the Capital of Arkansas gave me a
bit of trouble. During this whole year I was encouraged
and stimulated by a running fire of sarcasm from my
numerous relatives—all, that is, except my mother, who
stood by me without a word once her mind had been made
up. At the time I was very bitter about these Job's com-
forters of mine. Now I know that they kept me so angry
that they unintentionally furnished me with the added
incentive I needed. At the end of this year of cramming I

passed the Regents' examinations, packed my bag and set out on my rather lonely great adventure. I knew that I had finally left my home and that I would never go back except for short visits. It was hardly comforting knowledge, but I could not let anyone know how little confidence I felt in myself or the possibility of my ever justifying the expenditure of that precious $5,000.

In selecting the Women's Medical College of the New York Infirmary, only because I knew of no other place to go, I had unwittingly put myself into direct contact with the fountainhead of all medical training for American women. On the third of February, 1821, in Bristol, England, Elizabeth Blackwell was born, the third daughter in a family of nine children. In August, 1832, the entire Blackwell family set out on the seven weeks' voyage to America. Elizabeth Blackwell was the first woman in modern times to be graduated in medicine and to receive the degree of M.D. (1849) and she was the first woman doctor to be placed on the British Medical Register (1859). She died in Kilmun, England, in 1910. She spent her early years teaching in America, in order to earn the money to carry out her long-conceived plan of studying medicine, and then made application to as many medical colleges as she could reach for this opportunity. The idea of a woman studying medicine was abhorrent to all of them. The answers to her request were invariably, emphatically "No." Some friend of hers suggested her writing to a small medical college in Geneva, New York, and in October, 1847, she received a letter from the Dean of the Faculty of Geneva University telling her that her proposal had been submitted to the students who, acting independently and without any interference on the part of the Faculty, had invited her to join them. I feel that this resolution, opening as it did the medical profession to women students, is of such importance that it should be reproduced here:

At a meeting of the entire medical class of Geneva Medical College held this day, October 20th, 1847, the following resolutions were unanimously adopted:—

1. *Resolved*—That one of the radical principles of a Republican Government is the universal education of both sexes; that to every branch of scientific education the door should be open equally to all; that the application of Elizabeth Blackwell to become a member of our class meets with our entire approbation; and in extending our unanimous invitation we pledge ourselves that no conduct of ours shall cause her to regret her attendance at this institution.

2. That a copy of these proceedings be signed by the Chairman and transmitted to Elizabeth Blackwell.

T. J. STRATTON, *Chairman**

On January 23, 1849, Elizabeth Blackwell received her degree, and to her every medical woman owes a debt of gratitude. After several years of graduate study in this country, England and France, Dr. Blackwell decided that other women must have the opportunity that she had earned for them. Her efforts to establish a private practice in New York City were more than difficult. Women passing her in the street held their skirts aside so that they would not be contaminated by touching her. She has stated that her early practice was very much a Quaker practice and the colony of Quakers in New York supported her during these trying early years and made possible the founding of the New York Infirmary. I am proud to be one of this grand sect. Elizabeth's sister, Emily Blackwell,

* *Pioneer Work*, by Dr. Elizabeth Blackwell. E. P. Dutton & Co. New York.

was graduated from the Medical College of Cleveland in 1854, and in 1856 these two pioneer women together with Dr. Marie E. Zackrzewska, who had also just graduated from the Cleveland college, rented a house at 64 Bleecker Street and opened it as a dispensary where women physicians could get the opportunities for clinical work denied them at other places. It was named "The New York Infirmary for Women and Children." Later it was incorporated under this name and a medical college for women was also incorporated as part of its teaching plan. This was the college I had entered.

Dr. Emily Blackwell was at the head of this college in my day. Her sister, Dr. Elizabeth, had gone back to England to do her part in opening equal opportunities for English women. Dr. Zackrzewska had gone to Boston to be instrumental in opening a hospital where women physicians could obtain their needed graduate work. I was later an interne at this hospital—the New England Hospital for Women and Children. A group of women in Philadelphia, in 1850, opened a medical college for women in that city and today, with almost universal co-educational opportunities for women wishing to study medicine, this latter is the only strictly medical college-for-women-only still in existence.

Dr. Emily Blackwell, in her personality and appearance as well as in her achievements, belonged to the tradition of the great pioneers. She inspired us all with the vital feeling that we were still on trial and that, for women who meant to be physicians, no educational standards could be too high. It was a real advantage to be trained under that tradition. Years afterward, one night at a dinner, I sat next to Dr. William H. Welch, the much honored and greatly loved Dean of Johns Hopkins School of Hygiene and

Public Health. He confided to me that he had once belonged to the small group of medical men who prepared the examination questions for the students of the Women's Medical College. "And," he said, "I am now ashamed of the type of question we required those young women to answer. I am sure no one would have tolerated them in our own colleges. But our excuse must be that Dr. Blackwell demanded more difficult questions than could be submitted to our students, for she was determined that all women graduated from her college should be a carefully selected group."

I think that determination was clear all through our course. The New York Infirmary Medical College was the first to establish a chair for the teaching of hygiene. In 1859, it appointed a "sanitary visitor" whose duty it was "to give simple, practical instruction to poor mothers on the management of infants and the preservation of the health of their families." It was one of the earliest hospitals to establish a training school for nurses, and was the second medical college in the United States to require a four-year course before graduation—the first was Harvard University. In fact, all through those first years, not only were the highest standards maintained but the pioneering spirit persisted. I think not many of us realized that we were going out into the world as test cases, but Dr. Blackwell did. Later I realized the wisdom and extent of her vision.

I wish I might paint an adequate word-portrait of Dr. Emily Blackwell as I remember her. Tall, broad-shouldered and commanding in her presence, she was a striking figure, but I think few of us thought much about her general appearance. It was her face and her head that arrested your attention. I dislike to use the word "noble" in a physical description but it is the only adequate way to portray her face. Her hair was white when I knew her, and her whole personality was so striking and dominant that when she entered a room full of students, there suddenly seemed to be only one person in that room and that person was Dr. Blackwell. I never knew Dr. Elizabeth but I count it a great honor to have known Dr. Emily. Her voice was low and calm and of an uncanny quality: you could have heard the proverbial pin drop in any room where she was speaking. She looked into the future with prophetic clarity, and her great wisdom was nowhere more evident than when, one year after my own graduation, in 1899, she decided that a separate medical school for women was no longer necessary. In that year Cornell University established its medical school in New York City and, by the terms of its University Charter, it had to be co-educational. That was the first opportunity, in New York City, for women to work with men on equal terms, and Dr. Blackwell sensed its importance. She decided that the goal for which she and Dr. Elizabeth had worked was at last achieved: women must compete with and work with men in the medical profession. The day of separate education was over. From that time on a women's medical college would retard rather than advance the best interests of women and so, after arrangements had been made for all of the students to be entered in their respective classes at Cornell, the college closed its doors.

When I think back to those years so long ago, it is difficult to keep a proper sequence in mind. The idea of women in the medical profession is so familiar and commonplace to me now, and it was so strange and unconventional then. Possibly, my life should have been romantically exciting but I didn't find it so. It was half terrifying and half bor-

ing for the first few months. I was not quite eighteen but
quite old enough to worry over the time and money I
might be wasting if I did not succeed. The other members
of my class of thirty-five students seemed older and rather
remote. Even the plodding and elementary work of learning the names of muscles and bones, trying to get some
sane idea of elementary physiology and equally elementary
chemistry, which were the starting points, did not wholly
occupy my mind. I had too much spare time and nothing
to do with it and only the chorus of "I told you so's" which
would have greeted me kept me from dropping it all and
going home.

Sometimes I sat brooding in Stuyvesant Square, which
was then a quiet place with many flower-beds. Sometimes
I sat in Union Square which was also a quiet place and
aeons removed from the Communistic stamping ground
and noisy, barren annex to Klein's that it is now. But I
soon found out that the best way to kill spare time was to
climb up on the driver's seat of one of the old Fifth Avenue horse-drawn busses, ride up to the car barns at Eighty-
fourth Street and then, when the horses had been changed,
ride back again. It would take all of an afternoon or an
evening to make this trip. The busses were queer old
vehicles. Inside they had long seats on either side seating
possibly twelve or fourteen people. There was a little
slotted opening up in the room in front and through this
one put his quarter or fifty-cent piece and in time the
driver would push back an envelope with the printed in-
scription: "Change for twenty-five cents," or "fifty cents."
If you had the right change with you, your dime went
into a glass contraption in the front of the bus and a bell
rang to vouch for your honesty in paying your fare. But
the seat outside with the driver was the vantage point.

There was room for three people in all but, as it required a good deal of athletic prowess to climb up, it was reserved for the elect. The drivers of those days are now an extinct race—they have disappeared as have the old-time London busmen—but while they lasted they had a flavor and quality of language, and of information too, that made them rare and illuminating companions for a lonely girl.

Fifth Avenue is now completely altered; in my early days it was solidly filled with brownstone houses, of varying sizes but with an appalling uniformity for all that. The driver knew who lived in each one and had anecdotes galore to fit the different families. I knew a few of these families myself but had sworn a solemn vow that there were to be no social contacts in my new life, so I neither went to see them nor let them know that I was in town as a medical student. From Twenty-third Street to Fifty-ninth Street there were no shops; just the tightly closed houses of what was then the traditional residence district of Ward McAllister's "Four Hundred." Famous names and huge fortunes came from the driver's mouth to the accompaniment of the rattle of the bus wheels on the cobblestone pavement. Down each side-street stretched double rows of brownstone houses with high stoops, all exactly alike—at once dismal and charming in the bright autumn sunlight or the early gas-light of the evening. Everything leisurely and solid. That was not the same New York I came to know later, the New York of hurrying politics and crowded tenements. The old reservoir—looking like a mediaeval fortification—still covered the block at Forty-second Street where the public library now stands. Above Fifty-ninth Street great new mansions in the lavish pre-war style were building, but most of them were flanked on both sides by vacant lots.

Several times each week I would spend the afternoon or evening at Proctor's Vaudeville Theatre on West Twenty-third Street. Some weeks I went every day seeing the same show over seven times before it changed at the end of the week. You have to be either very lonesome or terribly fond of vaudeville to endure such an ordeal. I was both. But the people near me would probably have been startled to know that the small and shrinking young girl next them, wearing a street-sweeping skirt and an elaborately feathered hat, like everyone else, was nursing a bag of human bones in her lap all the time the comedians were going through their hilarious acts on the stage. Bones are the breath of life to the first-year medical student and I usually carried my collection with me, as a Chinese Mandarin carries his favorite bit of jade, to mull over them and attach imaginary muscles to them at odd moments.

I lived in a boarding house in West Seventeenth Street between Fifth and Sixth Avenues. It filled several houses thrown together and offered very little in social contacts. But there were a few isolated young men and women like myself there, all with little enough money and all starting out to carve their respective ways in the world. Most of them became very successful and some of them wealthy— a typical American start and finish. We used to pool our resources and go to as many plays as the money allowed. Boarding houses, which were common enough at that time, seem to have almost entirely disappeared. They offered a refuge for the unattached young man or young woman and for young married couples without enough money to start housekeeping on their own. There were always a few much older people, couples usually, who had not been treated too well by time, and to them the boarding house was a haven of refuge. They were often dull places and

the food was the subject of constant witticisms and jokes
but I cannot think that there is now any sufficient substitute for all that they offered. Today, these people would
be living isolated in small apartments on intimate terms
with the can-opener. But in the eighteen-nineties the
modern apartment house was still in an embryonic stage.
About the only social occasion I remember with much
vividness out of that first year is being at a party which
included the famous Julia Ward Howe; a very impressive
and delightful old lady. Some one asked her to recite *The
Battle Hymn of the Republic,* and I have a very clear picture of Mrs. Howe arising from her chair and giving us
that immortal hymn. It gave me a never-to-be-forgotten
impression of its grandeur. Ever since, I have been chron-
ically unable to understand why it should not be the American national anthem. It is not only that the words are far
more impressive than those of *The Star Spangled Banner,*
but the tune is superb, far more singable, and a native
American product. But then I suppose the American nation would have to have a national anthem beginning
"Oh, say . . . ."

My fellow-students at the College not only were older
than I was, with few exceptions, but they were seriously
absorbed in their work. There was little feminine consciousness apparent. The student who asked me to subscribe
to a suffrage paper was the only one who ever showed signs
of that future fever. There was nothing for me to do but
to get absorbed in work too. I managed that fairly grace-
fully and gradually the homesickness and the loneliness
disappeared and I found myself becoming intensely interested and busy as the real meaning of the course of study
began to emerge. Dissecting, which proved to be strangely
impersonal, threatened to be a difficult hurdle to scale, but

actually it never worried me and from that time I was heart and soul bound by the interest and fascination of it all. Gradually I began to make friends. Five of them are still my friends, though I do not see them now as often as I should like: Dr. Caroline H. LeFevre who became a highly successful surgeon, Dr. Marie Louise Lefort who has been for many years at the head of the American Hospital at Rheims, France, Dr. Alice Asserson with whom I worked in the Children's Welfare Federation for many years, Dr. Lillian K. P. Farrar who has achieved distinction as the only woman staff surgeon in a man-staffed hospital in New York City and who has a record of distinction that may well be envied by any medical man or woman, and Dr. Florence M. Laighton with whom I lived and practiced for many years. All splendid women who, even in their student days, were marked for future success.

But even more important than such fertile association with potentially first-class doctors was the general training in sound, shrewdly acquired knowledge. That was implicit in everything that happened—sometimes gradually and solemnly, sometimes ironically. For instance, in my student days I was one of those people who liked to suspect that most inhabitants of insane asylums are as sane as those outside and that, in many cases, scheming relatives or people unwilling to be bothered by the more eccentric kind of human being used the asylum as an unjustified answer to selfish impulses. On one occasion, when we students were going through an insane asylum, I went out of my way to mention to one of the resident physicians that the inmates looked and sounded quite as sane as I was.

"You do get that impression," he said. "If you want to try it out—well, choose anybody you like and talk to him and give me your opinion on him. But mind you, you must talk to him at least ten minutes before you make up your mind."

I chose my man—a quiet, easy-mannered individual to whom I found myself talking as sanely and conventionally as if I had just met him at a social party. He spoke of this and that and then asked me to get in touch with a certain person "outside" who would make a real effort to get him out, if only his plight could be properly represented. I wrote down the address of the "outside" person very carefully and listened while the inmate explained just how he had been railroaded into the asylum.

"But," I asked, "why did they want to treat you that way?"

"Ah," he said, "that's the story. They wanted to get my invention out of my hands."

"Your invention?" I asked.

"Yes," he said, "it'll make their fortunes. It's the greatest thing since the steam-engine. I have invented and perfected the wonder of the age—a paper lining for lamp-chimneys, to make them easier to clean."

Perhaps that is a little too farcical to be real irony. But irony is certainly present in the fact that the one subject I failed in medical school was to be the foundation of my life-work. This was related to a course, during my sophomore year, on "The Normal Child," given by Dr. Annie Sturges Daniel, a pioneer woman physician who is loved and honored by every student who came under her influence. Dr. Daniel's course was an uncharted sea and I had no interest in it; neither had anyone else so far as I could discover except Dr. Daniel herself. No other college had such a course and anything normal seemed far removed from the subjects that medical colleges had to teach in those days. There was, naturally, no textbook on the subject, with one minor exception which did not seem either interesting or informative. There were Dr. Daniel's lectures, to be sure, but they seemed to have little bearing upon the future career of a would-be doctor. It was a subject far in advance of the time and Dr. Daniel had practically invented it herself, believing as she did that no doctor could be reasonably intelligent about abnormal children until he, or she, knew what the normal child might be like. The intellectual soundness of that position left my callous young mind cold and disinterested and, as a result, I "flunked" that course because I had done no work in it at all.

That was my first, and only, failure. It not only gave a severe jolt to my pride but roused in me a fierce anger at having to take the course over again the following year. I made up my mind that, stupid as it might seem, I intended to learn all there was to know about the normal child. I took voluminous notes on the lectures; I read everything I could find that had the slightest relation to the subject, combing all the available libraries for scraps of information about that unusual phenomenon. The lectures, I discovered, once I started listening to them, were very fine; the bits of sought-out information most intriguing. As a result, that little pest, the normal child, made such a dent on my consciousness that it was he, rather than my lame knee, who is undoubtedly responsible for the survival of those 90,000 babies the reporter mentioned. The whole procedure of preventive hygiene which I was later to install in modern child care certainly had its inspiration in that half-year of pique and hard work. Everything that Dr. Daniel taught me in 1895 is still truer than ever in 1939. Neither she nor I had any idea that she was preparing me for thirty years of child welfare crusading. But, when the opportunity came, I was ready and eager for it and I, as well as the babies, owe a debt of gratitude to Dr. Daniel which I can never repay.

Some day, someone will write the epic story of the medical student. It will come from a doctor, of course, but it will be written, I think, by someone whose student days are far in the background. I am not the one, for it all seems very hazy and unreal to me now. I know there were four long years of grinding study, four years of irresponsible happiness, and four years so remote from the real work of the world that one might as well have been in a convent.

Many among those who taught me stand out in my memory: Dr. Gertrude B. Kelly, the friend of all lost causes, whose personal charm and beauty made her seem like a shy young girl and who yet contrived to be such a valiant fighter for the underdog that, when I spoke at her funeral a few years ago, I found my fellow speakers were representatives of the fighting Irish, determined Jews, radicals of all degrees, ex-prisoners for political so-called "crimes," and even atheists—all loving her and all proud to be called her friends. I remember one day when she had a friend call me over the telephone to tell me she was in jail, arrested for blocking Fifth Avenue traffic as she carried a huge banner calling attention to some social wrong, and asking me to go to Jefferson Market Court to act as a character witness for her. I found her as gay and amused as always. The charge was dismissed, but not until Dr. Kelly had whispered in my ear: "I loved being in jail. I was only there for three hours and I sold four thousand dollars' worth of Irish bonds to the other prisoners." She was a lovely soul. Among the others who made a definite imprint on my young mind, a few still stand out: Dr. Henry Mann Silver, Dr. George Roe Lockwood, Miss Chevalier—who could make even chemistry interesting,

Dr. Martha Wollstein, Dr. Alice Wakefield, Dr. Emily Lewi, Dr. Eleanor B. Kilham, and Dr. Elizabeth Cushier. There were hosts of others, to be sure, but these are the ones to whom I am most indebted.

At last, in the spring of 1898, my coveted diploma was given me. I was a real doctor at last—or so I thought then.

Chapter III

THE PRIVILEGE AND HONOR OF WRITING M.D. after his name is always a great spiritual comfort to the newly graduated medical student. It was a particular joy to me because so many inhabitants of Poughkeepsie had prophesied that I would never go through with it; and were now greeting the news that I had done so with rather scant appreciation. In spite of all the impressive Latin on the sheepskin, however, "M.D." in itself does not mean much. A student fresh out of medical school is no more a doctor than a man who has taught himself to go through swimming motions across a chair is a swimmer. That, of course, is why experience either as interne in a hospital or other graduate experience is almost an essential before beginning actual practice. The average year of routine interning may not teach you a great deal but it does clarify all that you have learned and give you the time and opportunity to turn theory into practice.

So I became an interne, addressed as Dr. Baker for the first time, wearing a white uniform and doing actual work in a hospital. Since I had graduated second in a class of eighteen (the rest of the thirty-five had fallen by the wayside), I was offered a fine interneship in the New York Infirmary for Women and Children, the hospital in connection with the college where I had taken my degree. But I felt that I needed to cut away from this familiar environment, to which I had devoted four whole years, that I needed new associates and a new point of view. That idea took me to Boston where I applied for, and obtained, a position as interne in the New England Hospital for Women and Children. There was no question of getting into a large general hospital. At that time no such institution admitted women in any capacity. Strange as it may sound in this year of 1939, few enough of them have yet seen the light sufficiently to admit women.

Still, the New England Hospital fitted my needs admirably. It was staffed entirely by women of first-rate calibre. The superintendent of nurses was Miss Clara Noyes who, when she died last year, was superintendent of nurses of the American Red Cross. It provided a wide range of medical, surgical and obstetrical work, which is always the best possible training for an interne. I grew very keen about surgery now that I had an opportunity of meeting its problems; it is clean, definite work with visible results and a consciousness of direct accomplishment. When you remove an appendix or amputate a leg you have done the indicated thing for good and all, whereas, in handling medical cases, at best, it is a matter of being a watchman always and the help one can give, with the best intentions in the world, must vary. If I had been exposed to the modern cult for specialization, I should probably have become a woman-surgeon, several of whom have made great names for themselves. I have great sympathy with and understanding of the fact that the majority of medical students make surgery their goal. But as it was, I thought of nothing beyond preparing myself for general practice and of making up sleep on that half-day a week when an interne was not on call. There was little question of amusement during one's time off; both energy and money were lacking.

Part of our service was three months of duty in the out-

practice department. We spent this time in a completely
equipped clinic in Fayette Street, Boston, which served a
huge poverty-stricken clientele drawn from among the
inhabitants of Boston's worst slums, which were quite as
bad as any in the country at that time. This was hard work
and, when your financial resources were as slim as mine
were, you got little enough nourishment for fuel to do it
on. Each interne was given four dollars a week to feed
herself. Things were cheaper then than now, but even so
we were in no danger of over-eating. Dr. Florence Laighton, a fellow interne, and I went in on a system to make it
last as long as possible. Six days a week we ate at the Y. W.
C. A., which cost three dollars, largely for indeterminate
stews, baked beans, bread and stewed prunes. I really have
not cared for beans since. Then, on Sunday, when we were
both certain that we could not stand this kind of fare any
longer, we would spend our remaining dollar apiece and
have one good meal at the old Thorndike Hotel which
would help us to survive until the following Sunday.

That was only one of the ways in which I had now to
adjust myself to a kind of reality of which I had never
dreamed at home, or at medical school either. For the first
time in my life I was really up against facts. No student,
whether in law or medicine, is living a real life. An academic atmosphere is necessarily artificial. Here, in Boston,
submerged in the hectic life of a big clinic, I was abruptly
forced to translate what I had studied into actuality, to
realize that the luridly colored pictures in ponderous medical texts meant actual fever and pain and delirium and
mutilation, and that those crisp summaries of what to do
about this or that physical ailment, which had sounded so
reassuring on the printed page, were of distressingly little
help to an inexperienced beginner. It was all the more dis-

couraging because the raw material we worked with on Fayette Street was anything but pretty. We were dealing with the dregs of Boston, ignorant, shiftless, settled irrevocably into surly degradation. Just to make sure they would be hopeless, many of them drank savagely. Having borne children and lived and fought and made love regardless, they took that method of dodging the consequences. Nothing admirable about it, but one could not honestly blame them for making use of alcohol as an anaesthetic.

In time I got used to it, if not hardened to it. But, for the first few weeks at the clinic, my inexperienced and still reasonably girlish soul was aghast at the discovery that, with these people, any and every calamity was such a matter of course. There was the Irishwoman who came to the Hospital to be delivered of a baby. She looked much too old for motherhood, but then you get wrinkled and bent quickly under the conditions she had always known. On admission she proved to have both feet badly burned in addition to her other difficulties. I asked her how the burns happened. "Well, deary," she said, "I come in a night or two ago with me feet wet and I stuck thim in the oven to dry thim and forgot thim." Drunk, no doubt, drifting peacefully off into an alcoholic fog with a new life in her waiting to be born, and much too numb to know that her feet were blistering in the oven. Numb—that seems to be the right word for all of them.

Presently I signalized my new acquaintance with reality by committing murder—to all intents and purposes. That came about with appalling naturalness. It was another obstetrical case, a routine hurry call to come to a woman who was about to have a baby. A man with a long beard brought the message. He silently guided me through snow-choked alleyways to an old frame house hidden in a court.

As soon as he saw me started up to the top floor, he went away; I had the idea that he was afraid to accompany me for some reason. But I went on up the stairs, feeling with my feet for loose boards and holes in the enveloping darkness, and found my patient at last.

I thought I already knew something about how filthy a tenement room could be. But this was something special, particularly in the amount of insect life. One dingy oil lamp, by the light of which I could barely make out the woman in labor, lying on a heap of straw in one corner. Four stunted children, too frightened to make any noise, huddled together in a far corner. The floor was littered with scraps of food, too old to be easily identifiable, but all contributing to the odor of the place. Cockroaches and bedbugs crawled about everywhere. The only thing to wash up in was, as usual, an old tin basin, rusted and ragged at the edge. All of it was the nth power of abject, discouraged squalor. But the ugliest detail was a man, also lying on the floor because he was apparently too drunk to get up. But he was all too capable of speech.

The moment I approached my patient I discovered that her back was one raw, festering sore. She said that her husband had thrown a kettle of scalding water over her a few days before. That accusation brought him to his feet crazy with rage, threatening me and her, toppling and lurching all over the place.

I knew that could not go on. I had to get him out of the way. As he wavered toward me, waving his clenched fist and uttering verbal filth, I ran out into the hall. He followed as I had intended. I had thought of running in quickly again and seeing if the door would lock. But then, as he lurched after me, he crossed the stair-head and, with instinctive reaction, I doubled my fist and hit him.

It was beautifully timed. I weighed hardly half as much as he, but he was practically incapable of standing up, and this frantic tap of mine was strategically placed. He toppled backward, struck about a third of the way down the rather long stair and slid to the bottom with a hideous crash. Then there was absolute silence. I had taken my opportunity and the result was evident. I went back into the room, pushed a piece of furniture against the closed door and delivered the baby undisturbed.

Under stress of this emergency work, I did not have much time to speculate on what had happened to my victim. Only when the delivery was finished, the room partly cleaned up, the children cared for and the patient made relatively comfortable, did I collect my wits enough to start meditating on the fact that I had probably killed a man. I suppose it should have sickened me with anxiety but I was too tired to make emotional sense of the situation. It had been sheer reflex instinct; he was in the way and not fit to live anyhow and I had taken the first handy means of getting rid of him. I was not sorry; I was not glad either—it had just been part of the exigencies of this particular job. Well, I thought, as calmly as I could, there is the end of your medical career and probably jail to follow.

By the time I reached the head of the stairs on my way out, however, I did comprehend that the body was down in the hall and that something probably ought to be done about it. So I went and knocked at a door across the hall. A man appeared, half dressed, apparently too sleepy to be startled by my telling him that I had killed his next door neighbor. He just said "humph" and went downstairs with me to find out what it was all about. There was the body lying motionless as I expected, crumpled against the wall where it had struck head-foremost. My escort scowled and gave it a kick in the ribs. It still did not move. But it did emit a gust of bass profanity which was the sweetest sound I ever heard in my life. Only then, when I realized that he was not dead, did I fully realize what it would have meant to have killed him. I think that in those relatively few moments I did more growing up than I had done in my previous twenty-odd years.

At the end of our year as internes, Dr. Laighton and I went back to New York to seek what advice we could get about the chance of our starting to practice in that city. Our old professors at the medical college, our acquaintances among established practitioners, all said the same thing: "If you have enough money to support yourselves for five years entirely and for another five years in part, you stand a fighting chance in New York. If you haven't, New York is hopeless. Go to some small town and do the best you can." In my case only a few hundreds remained of the $5,000 I had taken from my father's estate. Dr. Laighton was little better off. The obvious thing was to return to Poughkeepsie where being well known would give me a favorable start. But I liked New York; I have always liked it in spite of its noise, its confusion and its seeming indifference. We had the usual resiliency of youth and we discarded this wise advice. We thanked all of our advisers and rented an apartment on West Ninety-first Street, near Central Park, took a few weeks off to pass our State Regents' examinations, hung out our shingles and, with inexplicable equanimity, had no fear at all for the future. Dr. Laighton's family gave us enough money to furnish the place and equip our office and we had every intention of staying. It was just imbecile optimism. The advice we had received was all too sound. I would give it myself in about the same words to any young doctors who asked me what to do nowadays. And they would probably refuse to act upon it just as we did.

Paradoxically, our only asset was that we were women doctors. We were almost the only ones established on the west side of New York above Fifty-ninth Street. For many years women came to us because we were women and the competition in that line was small. But we deserved to starve and I do not know why we did not. My first year's proceeds amounted to exactly $185.00. And, except that I was paid for it, my first case was a sample of the whole year. In those days, Amsterdam Avenue, which has since experienced both a feverish building-boom and a period of gradual decline, was filled with squatters' shacks made of hammered-out tin cans and waste lumber, inhabited by ne'er-do-wells and swarming with goats. I began my practice by delivering a baby in one of those shacks. Again it was a hurry call and they had sent for me much too late; it was a difficult and abnormal case. Even with Dr. Laighton's assistance, saving the mother and keeping the baby alive for an hour or two was the best I could do. But the father gave me ten dollars, which considering his economic necessities, was extremely decent of him.

Obstetrics have been a godsend to many a young doctor just starting his career. It is the one sure event in medicine, for babies are always with us. It is an opening wedge of considerable importance to have an obstetric case, stay on as the baby's doctor and then, when in the natural order of events the father or mother comes down with a cold or some other minor ailment, to find that you are consulted and have other patients. It was in this way that my practice was built up and became a truly family affair. A not too prosperous, but not too poverty-stricken neighborhood with a fairly high birthrate seems to me an ideal place for the struggling young physician to make his start.

A dollar bill should have been saved out of that first ten, to frame and hang in my office. But that was economically impossible. A dollar was such a rare object. On one occasion when I was down to my last two dollars in the world, I defiantly spent it on a grand lunch at the old Waldorf Hotel and a magazine to read on the trolley car going home. Rent day was just around the corner too. But when I reached our apartment, there was a patient waiting who paid me in cash and enabled me to carry on a little longer. Our economic status in those days and our ability to carry on will always remain as a great mystery to me. Somehow, we always did manage and we never got into debt. I suppose that proves something, but just what I frankly do not know.

Being young, we were incapable of worrying. But we did have to use our mother-wit to find ways of supplementing our incomes. For that purpose a call from a much too persistent life-insurance agent proved accidentally helpful. In order to get rid of him, we asked if the company had a woman doctor to examine us if we did take out insurance. He said no, certainly not—he had never heard of such a thing. Our tones were shocked as we said that we would never think of being examined by a man doctor and we showed him to the door with well-simulated indignation. Then, after he was gone, it occurred to us that many women might think as we did and that it would be a sound scheme for the insurance companies to have women-examiners on call.

Having plenty of time in which to pursue the idea, Dr. Laighton and I went down town the next day, she to visit

the New York Life Insurance Company while I went to the
Equitable. Each of us had the same experience. In both
places the Chief Medical Examiner was mildly amused at
the idea. But we went on stubbornly pointing out the advantages in the scheme and eventually persuaded the companies to inform their agents that, when a prospective
client wanted one, a woman examiner would be available
in our persons. We came away enrolled as special medical
examiners. That brainstorm of ours brought us a steady
stream of profitable fees and opened up that whole field of
medical activity for women. I hope that our successors have
found it as profitable as we did. One day I was sent up to
West End Avenue to examine a client and much to my
surprise met Lillian Russell there. She was a truly great
and beautiful woman. I was always an inveterate theater-
goer, until my public health work made me too busy to
take more than a very occasional evening off for the
theater, so I stayed chatting with her for most of the afternoon. She was the loveliest, most natural and most charming person I had ever seen and there have been few to
match her since. It was one of my first red-letter days.

I was in general practice for a number of years. But as
events turned out, private practice was not to be my whole
career and after fifteen years of dividing my interests, it
was inevitable that it should be discarded. I was hardly
well started when another accident, the mere catching
sight of an item in the morning paper, diverted me into
taking the first step toward my real career. The paper said
that civil service examinations for the postion of medical
inspector of the Department of Health would be held at
such a time and place; the salary to be thirty dollars a
month. A dollar a day: about double my first year's rate
of income. It was tempting enough to make me take the

[54]

examination and I came out high enough on the passed list
for a possible appointment. Ordinarily I would have supposed that this would guarantee me the job. But by this
time I was vaguely aware that there was corruption in city
politics and that people sometimes had to use pull to get
city appointments. That really was the innocent extent of
my knowledge of what I was getting into. So I asked a
lawyer patient of mine to give me a letter of recommendation to a justice of the New York Supreme Court who was,
of course, right in the middle of politics and the justice
passed me on with another letter to one of the, then, three
Commissioners of Health. R. A. Van Wyck was then the
Mayor and not until the succeeding administration of
Mayor Seth Low did the Department function under its
present plan of one commissioner.

The Department headquarters were at that time in a
forlorn old building at the corner of Sixth Avenue and
Fifty-fifth Street which had formerly housed the New
York Athletic Club and had obviously been neither cleaned
nor painted since the athletes had vacated it. As the central
focus of the sanitary and medical services of a great city,
it was a shock; the Commissioner was another. I do not
remember his name, but he could have sat as a cartoon for
the public idea of a typical Tammany henchman. He was
paunchy with a fat blue-jowled face and sat with his feet
on the desk, his hat on the back of his head and the last two
inches of a disorganized cigar in the corner of his mouth.
I had supposed he would ask me some questions but he did
not deign to do that. He did not even look at me twice. He
just opened my letter, glanced through it, rang a bell and,
when a clerk appeared, he jerked his thumb at me over his
shoulder and said: "Give the lady her appointment." That
was my first lesson in the ways of the world of I'll-do-you-

a-favor-sometime. It was also my launching in public health work.

Inspecting school children was my first assignment and it seemed to me to be a pathetic farce. We inspectors went around to certain assigned schools and asked the teachers if any pupils showed any signs of illness. If, by chance, a teacher had noticed that a child did not seem well, we looked him over, more or less perfunctorily, and sent him home if we suspected some form of contagious disease. There was not, and could not be, any serious attempt at diagnosis. Our appointment was for one hour's work a day and in that time we had to visit three or four schools. Another inspector was sent to visit the child at home and decide whether or not he was to be excluded from school. But, in view of some later discoveries of mine, there is fairly good reason to doubt that this follow-up proved much. The only thing to recommend the whole dismal business was that it did, in a futilely primitive fashion, recognize that something might conceivably be done about controlling contagious diseases in school children.

I stayed away from the Department office except on pay-day. I could not stand the atmosphere of the place, either literally or figuratively. It reeked of negligence and stale tobacco smoke and slacking. It was inconceivable that any such organization could accomplish more than merely keeping a certain number of political hangers-on firmly attached to the public payroll. Many inspectors, as I learned later, never bothered to go to their schools at all, merely making the concession of telephoning each school each morning. Yet no one bothered to call them to account. In honest moments, I could not help feeling that my own job was a minor racket too, for, even if I did work at it, I knew that I was accomplishing no good whatever. But that dollar a day came in very handily and I decided to stay until summer when, with the closing of the schools, I felt that this temporary adventure into the political field would be over.

In the end I was glad that I had stayed. When Mayor Seth Low came into office in 1902 and Dr. Ernst J. Lederle was appointed Commissioner of Health, the whole department shuddered at the shake-up and house-cleaning that occurred. At the beginning, I knew little or nothing of that for I had no interest in the administrative side of my job. But I did know that in the shaking-up process I was sent for by a new assistant sanitary superintendent and offered a summer position in hunting out and looking after sick babies. This new appointee, Dr. Walter Bensel, my chief for years afterwards, was about the only reason I had yet seen for changing my opinion of the Health Department and its works. He had every appearance of being energetic, clean-cut and honest; all of which proved true and all of which was a novelty. I liked him, and his attitude, so much that I changed my mind and took the offered job at an increase in salary to one hundred dollars a month.

This time I had let myself in for a really gruelling ordeal. Summer anywhere in New York City is pretty bad. In my district, the heart of old Hell's Kitchen on the west side, the heat, the smells, the squalor made it something not to be believed. Its residents were largely Irish, incredibly shiftless, altogether charming in their abject helplessness, wholly lacking in any ambition and dirty to an unbelievable degree. At the upper edge of Hell's Kitchen, just above Fifty-ninth Street, was the then largest colored district in town. Both races lived well below any decent level of subsistence. My job was to start in this district every morning at seven o'clock, work until eleven, then return for two hours more—from four to six. I climbed stair after stair, knocked on door after door, met drunk after drunk, filthy mother after filthy mother and dying baby after dying baby. It was the hardest physical labor I ever did in my life: just backache and perspiration and disgust and discouragement and aching feet day in and day out.

I worked out one minor way to save myself by going up the long flights of stairs to the roof of one tenement and then climbing the dividing wall to go down the stairs of the next. Trailing street-sweeping skirts were not much of a help. There was no dodging the hopelessness of it all. It was an appalling summer too, with an average of fifteen hundred babies dying each week in the city; lean, miserable, wailing little souls carried off wholesale by dysentery. Even New York's worst slums have now forgotten what dysentery epidemics were like. But we knew thirty years ago. The babies' mothers could not afford doctors and seemed too lackadaisical to carry their babies to the nearby clinics and too lazy or too indifferent to carry out the instructions you might give them. I do not mean that they were callous when their babies died. Then they cried like mothers, for a change. They were just horribly fatalistic about it while it was going on. Babies always died in summer and there was no point in trying to do anything about it. It depressed me so that I branched out and went looking for healthy babies too and tried to tell their mothers how to care for them. But they were not interested. I might as well have been trying to tell them how to keep it from raining.

One fantastic incident will illustrate their shiftlessness. A dead baby always meant a neat little white funeral because, no matter how poor the family were, they always insured their babies and usually received twenty-five dollars when the baby died—enough to pay for a cheap white coffin and a few wilted flowers. One afternoon, when I found a despairing family sitting around a baby's coffin in a stifling, cockroach-ridden room without a single cent to buy food, I let my feelings get the better of me and handed them a five dollar bill. A week later one of that family's numerous children showed up at my office and presented me with a cheap little photograph of one of the dead baby's survivors. "Mama always wanted a picture of one of us," she said gleefully, "but until you gave her that five dollars she had never had enough money to have one taken." Well, I suppose there must be hyacinths to feed one's soul.

Why I stayed on that job is another mystery. But I actually refused my regular summer laboratory work at the Dansville Sanitarium in order to stay with this brutal punishment. Perhaps the sight of such sluggish, crawling misery fascinated me. You could not say that I was sentimental about these people. I had a sincere conviction that they would all be better off dead than so degradingly alive. But they apparently had an instinct for life and I had to go through the motions of helping them. It did seem pretty futile. One could hardly walk a block in any tenement district in the city without meeting a "Little White Funeral." Dead horses (there were horses then) were a common sight in almost every street. Pasteurization of the milk supply was just beginning to be urged by that great philanthropist, Nathan Straus, but the bulk of the milk supply that these babies were fed on was drawn from rusty cans and the milk was dotted with flies as well as full of bacteria. One could do so little at best. In my mind was a vague idea that something could and must be done; what it might be I did not yet know, but I did know that it was infamous to let these things go on. I have heard out-of-towners ask the reason for Hell's Kitchen having that picturesque name. I could give them a good reason and it would not have anything to do with gangsters either.

Presently I was in such a frame of mind that no horror could be really disturbing. That was the summer of the *General Slocum* disaster, when an excursion boat filled with women and children on a picnic party burned in the East River and hundreds were drowned or burned. All of the Health Department inspectors were summoned by telephone to rush to North Brother Island, where bodies were being washed ashore from the burning vessel. There was precious little to do by the time we got there; it was just a question of getting the bodies out of the water and ranging them in long rows on the shore, dead woman after dead woman, dead child after dead child, all huddled and wet and still. It was fearful, I suppose, but you cannot realize things wholesale that way, any more than you could psychologically afford to realize the mass of misery in my Hell's Kitchen slum.

In fact one of my brother-inspectors was so little affected by the spectacle that while we were talking together on the ferry boat bringing us back from the island he chose to let me know that he, and a number of other inspectors, were finding my behavior thoroughly unethical.

"Do you realize," he asked me, "how tough you are making this job for the rest of us?"

I hope I looked as puzzled as I felt.

"I mean," he said, "you are spoiling things. You are actually inspecting tenements and reporting sick babies, aren't you?"

I admitted it.

[60]

"Well," he said, "I guess you just don't know any better. The boys asked me to tip you off. You don't need to go to all of that trouble. All we do is to ask the janitor how many families are in the building and note down that many families visited and let it go at that." He looked at my face whose expression must have been sufficiently queer, and went on, "Ordinarily that would be just your business. But if we don't report any sick babies and you go ahead and report shoals of them, it makes our reports look pretty bad. I thought you ought to know."

That was a problem. I had never aspired to be an Elsie Dinsmore; in fact I have never disliked anyone more than I do her. But I did know that there were at least a few other inspectors in the Department who really did work, honestly. The more I thought of it, the more I could see that this was a matter between me and the babies. I was truly puzzled. Did the Department really expect you to do your work, or didn't it? Was it all the same old racket?

And then things began to happen; I had been right about Dr. Bensel. He had been following the same line of reasoning as my fellow-inspector. It did not seem reasonable to him that dysentery should be confined to a few small slum districts surrounded by exactly similar districts which had not reported a single case. The storm broke and dozens of inspectors were dismissed. At last we were going to be honest and decent. At the end of the summer Dr. Bensel appointed me as his office assistant. Little as I liked getting my preferment that way, it was hardly a valid reason for refusing it. The cards had been dealt so and I could not have behaved otherwise.

I had long since acquired a burning sense of the injustice in the world, which was intensified by the conditions among these people with whom I had worked. My encounter with cynical dishonesty and resulting neglect of duty did not tend to reassure me. Without my knowing it, there was already shaping up in me the foundation of my whole active career—a career of struggling to force, persuade or cajole the social consciousness of the people to meet this challenge of the underworld.

This spectacle of official negligence, or worse, was the last straw I think. It was already horrible enough injustice that human machinery should always be in need of repair. The problems of food, clothing, shelter and children were in themselves almost too difficult to be solved. It did not seem fair that these people should have to cope with the results of official negligence and dishonesty. It was going to take a world of change to better all this; I knew that many people of many minds might ponder and work for generations before any change could be made in the social organism. I was only a raw beginner in the field of public health and all I had time or energy to realize was that the waste of life, at the beginning, might be prevented if only one knew how. For the moment, I could merely take bewilderedly to heart the one-sentence sermon preached to me by another drunken mother during my interne days in Boston.

This lady arrived late at night in a cab. An orderly rushed in to tell me that there was a "case" outside. Somewhere along the way, however, it had ceased to be a case. The baby was already born and lying on the cold cab floor, hidden under his mother's long skirts. The mother was so completely drunk that, so far as I could make out, she had experienced no discomfort at all during the baby's birth. With the nurse's help, we got her out, carried her into the hospital and placed her on a bed. She made no sound, just lay propped against a pillow with her hat over one eye, apparently quite oblivious of the fact that she had just brought another life into the world for good or ill. But, when I lifted the baby by the heels and spanked him in order to start him breathing, she did open her one visible eye. Its expression was the essence of that sad quizzicalness which seems to me to belong to the Irish more than to any other race:

"How unfortunate it is," she said, rolling it out like a preacher in a pulpit, "that, at the moment of our entrance into the world, we have to be chastised." Then having uttered that profound and really eloquently expressed sentiment, she fell back into an alcoholic slumber that lasted twenty-four hours.

CHAPTER IV

THE GIBSON GIRL WAS A GREAT HELP TO ME when I started work in the public health field. It is difficult to realize today how curious it seemed then that a woman should hold my position. A little later, when I was assistant to Dr. Darlington, the Commissioner of Health, they made me print my name on the letterheads as "Dr. S. J. Baker" to disguise the presence of a woman in a responsible executive post. The Gibson Girl played a part in the situation because, most fortunately for me, she had persuaded me and the world in general into accepting shirtwaists and tailored suits as a conventional feminine costume. I liked the effect and still do. But its convenience came in because, if I was to be the only woman executive in the New York City Department of Health, I badly needed protective coloring. As it was, I could so dress that, when a masculine colleague of mine looked around the office in a rather critical state of mind, no feminine furbelows would catch his eye and give him an excuse to become irritated by the presence of a woman where, according to him, no woman had a right to be. My man-tailored suits and shirtwaists and stiff collars and four-in-hand ties were a trifle expensive, but they more than paid their way as buffers. They were also very little trouble. I could order a suit and another dozen shirtwaists and collars with hardly a tenth of the time and energy that buying a single new frock would have required. And I had no time or energy to spare because, in the process of convincing myself that my work must be a success and equal to the best that might be done by a man in that man-made world, I invariably took home a brief case full of trouble every night and worked at it until the small hours of the morning. Dr. Mary Walker wore trousers to startle men into recognizing that a woman was demanding men's rights. I wore a standard costume—almost a uniform— because the last thing I wanted was to be conspicuously feminine when working with men. It all seems very strange now, for today women can be ultra-feminine and thus add attractiveness and charm to the work they are doing.

At home, of course, I kept a certain amount of conventional and thoroughly feminine attire for those rare occasions when I could allow myself a social holiday. And yet, I am sure that there are today a great number of my old-time friends who never saw me dressed in any other way, for I wore that costume in my daily work for over twenty-five years. When Commissioner Darlington gave a tea at the Plaza Hotel one day, I appeared in something rather frivolous for me. Several of the secretaries and clerks were there all dressed in their best. As I came in, I stopped for a word with two of the secretaries standing near the door. "Well, how's the party?" I asked. "Very nice," said one of them; "but to tell you the truth, doctor, we only came because we wanted to see whether you would wear a tailored suit and a stiff collar."

It seems queer too to think back those few years to the time when the world at large seemed genuinely convinced that women were not altogether bright. There are still probably many men who feel doubtful about taking orders from a woman, but women are now so generally accepted in the business and professional worlds that individually they get an opportunity of proving their worth before patronizing generalities begin to crop out. I had been at the head of the Bureau of Child Hygiene several years, I remember, when one day Dr. Alonzo Blauvelt started complaining to me about the appointment of some women doctors as medical inspectors. Women were all right in their way, he told me grievedly, but there was no getting around the fact that they were not trained to work in groups; they had no sense of cooperation, no idea of how to get the most out of their subordinates, no ability to take responsibility. I listened awhile, and then my sense of humor got the best of me. I laughed and said, "Now wait a minute, doctor. What kind of a creature do you think you are talking to now?" His jaw dropped and he blushed purple. "Good Lord," he said, "I'd entirely forgotten that you were a woman."

The modern young woman in the workaday world is a calm and efficient person who can take routine off the shoulders of her chief so that he can ponder matters of major policy and take two hours and a half over his lunch. There are thousands of her in the world of public and private management. At that time, a young woman in public life was as rare as a woman aviator and I had to take my job in male terms. And during those first few years I was a glorified jack-of-all-trades. There were the years in Dr. Bensel's office when I was sent out on unusual and always exciting assignments; the two years that I spent as an assistant to Dr. Herman M. Biggs, where Dr. William Studdiford and I had an opportunity of working out many public-health ideas. This was a rare experience. It gave me a background of the entire field of public health that made me decide then and there that it was a career. The rare wisdom of Dr. Biggs, coupled as it was with kindliness

and humanity, has left a memory that I shall always cher-
ish. I learned a great deal in those days: a range of information that ran from glanders in horses to tuberculosis
in man. We planned a campaign for the control of midwives that I later had a chance to put into effect, and the
first glimmer of an idea of what might be done to reduce
infant mortality on a large scale came to me then. I can
never be too grateful for those two years as a student of
Dr. Biggs'.

Then I was assigned to the office of Dr. Darlington and
given the official title of "Assistant to the Commissioner
of Health." And during nearly all of these years I was
what might be called a "trouble shooter." Anything which
did not fit into the assignments of the regular staff of inspectors fell to me. It was a fine idea. For one thing, it kept
life from anything like monotony. And for another, it
showed me that this field of public health was far removed
from anything that had been comprised in my conventional medical training. Not that medicine was not an
essential background—that was clear enough—but the
mass attack instead of individual care began to come to the
front. We were dealing with the problems of a community,
and the individual became important only when he con-
tributed to the problem as a whole.

And so the odds and ends of experience began to take
form in my eyes. There was a great deal that was rather
rough. Invading Bowery lodging-houses, the ten-cents-a-
night kind, for instance, to vaccinate the patrons against
small-pox in the very early hours of the morning. It had
to be done between midnight and six since the Bowery
floaters were up and away by the time dawn broke and
that was the only time to find them in any numbers. Few
of them were nature's noblemen, so I always had a Health

Department policeman by my side when I marched in; the usual picture being a huge, airless room in a decrepit old building that shook every time the elevated went by, filled with fully dressed men sleeping in musty blankets. The policeman would wake a man up and tell him to put out his arm. Then I would vaccinate him and pass on to the next. They were usually too far gone from bad whiskey to know very much about what was going on.

Things were exciting in another way when New York developed a spectacular and tragic epidemic of cerebrospinal meningitis and I became the temporary Department expert on the subject; not by merit, but because I happened to be the only member of the staff who had ever had much experience with this peculiarly horrible disease which then killed the majority of its victims and left the remainder maimed for life. Meningitis epidemics are fairly rare. While this one lasted I was dashing frantically all over New York, taking cultures, making spinal punctures, diagnosing and supervising cases and, in view of the patients' fearful sufferings, almost wishing that they would all be lucky enough to die. Noise and nuisance inspection were also thrown my way, which acquainted me with the perversities of insanitary plumbing—or no plumbing at all—smoke hazards and the filth of the overcrowded tenements that bred nuisances.

Since then New York has apparently decided to let the smoke nuisance get completely out of hand. In Dr. Darlington's administration, however, a black cloud pouring out of a chimney of a factory or an office building meant not only that the owner or operator was liable to arrest but that his employees must be taught how to stoke the furnaces so that this smoke could be prevented. New York had a clear atmosphere in those days; the smoke nuisance was controlled. Why it has been allowed to come back and why the health authorities are quiescent about this filthy nuisance, is one of the things that puzzle me today. As for noise, we had no noise at all in the modern sense. The screeching taxi-horn and the shouting radio had not yet been developed. But there were plenty of complaints, and in the intervals of writing pamphlets on rabies and the prevention of sunstroke and inspecting swimming pools and becoming the first editor of the Health Department's new Monthly Bulletin for the medical profession, I was assigned to nearly every variety of sanitary inspection.

There can hardly be an obscure corner of Manhattan Island into which I have not poked my official nose at one time or another. Sanitary conditions in New York City thirty years ago were far better than they had been in the fifties when chickens and pigs were running at large in the streets and the tenement houses, but by present-day standards conditions were pretty bad—just about as Jacob Riis described them in *How the Other Half Lives.* The lower east side of the city has been cleared out and cleaned up today; streets have been broadened and living-conditions improved to such an extent that it seems almost like a new world to me now. But thirty years ago the average tenement house that I visited was an ancient scandal, usually made up in the type of "railroad flats" of from two to four or five rooms in a continuous row with no hallway. Sometimes there would be one family to a room and too often there were boarders. Never a bathroom: that was unheard of. The better places had inside toilets; one to each floor. The older ones had outdoor privies in the backyard or court. The indoor privies were so filthy that I think the people with outdoor privies had slightly the better of it; at least these latter were cleaned out at night by a crew from the Department of Health. You might often find one room used as living-quarters by ten or a dozen people, taking it in shifts with some on night and some on day work. And a large section of the west side of the city was the same; all unutterably filthy and hopeless, particularly Hell's Kitchen. I grew to know this latter district well.

It was curious to see how conditions varied, depending upon the particular foreign colony you chanced to meet. The Germans were the cleanest; that was axiomatic. The Italians came next; not only would the front room of an Italian family usually be moderately clean but there would have been some pathetic attempt at brightening the place up with paper flowers, religious pictures and a fancy bedspread. It always amazed me to go into the big colored district, which was between Tenth Avenue and the river in the upper West Fifties then, instead of in Harlem as it is today. That district contained the densest population in town, with one block housing over six thousand people, but they managed to stay decent in spite of that inhuman handicap. The houses were clean in a sad poverty-stricken fashion and the children were kept so clean that I often wondered how it was done; they were always cheerful people too and I liked to work with them. The Irish and the Russian Jews vied for the distinction of living in the most lurid squalor. The Irish did it, as I already knew, out of a mixture of discouragement and apparent shiftlessness, but they were happy people too and soon pulled themselves up out of the ruck. They had an ambition that could survive almost anything. The Russian Jews did it out of thrift. Practically every Russian Jewish family had chosen one son who was to be supported through medical or law school as a way of raising the family fortune and prestige, and every penny that could be spared beyond the barest necessities of life was hoarded for that purpose. While Isador was being educated the whole family worked like mad under sweat-shop conditions and skimped incredibly on food, clothes and rent, not to mention soap and sunlight. Then when the chosen son started making money, they moved out and followed his rising fortunes uptown; first to Lexington Avenue, then to the Bronx, then to Riverside Drive and sometimes finally to Park Avenue or the upper East Fifties or Sixties. That was as regular a progression as spring, summer, autumn, winter. But again, I liked them too. They had not the gaiety of the Italians or the colored people but their ambition did get my respect.

The self-sufficiency of these Little Italys and these Little Ghettoes was incredible. The men went around a bit; they had to go to different parts of the town to work at their jobs. But the women ate, slept, cooked, washed and minded the baby strictly at home and did all the family buying at the pushcart in the immediate neighborhood. They had no curiosity and it never occurred to them to go outside of that necessary circle. In the years when the Health Department held Better Baby Contests, I went down on the East Side in a Department car to get a mother and her baby who were to be presented with a prize at a ceremony in Central Park. The mother stepped into the car remarking that she had never ridden in one before, which was understandable in 1910. But then she startled me by asking if perhaps she might be able to see a tree in this place to which she was going. She had been born and brought up under the approach to the Brooklyn Bridge and then moved, when she was married, to a tenement not far distant, evidently living all her life in shade so thick that not even the ailanthus trees, which will grow almost anywhere in New York's slum districts, could take root in her various backyards. Yet it was not that trees were inaccessible; there was a park full of trees only a few blocks from her street. It was just that she had never had any practical occasion to go that far away from home, so she never had.

The Italians were the cheeriest group as a rule. A call on an Italian family for any purpose whatever generally required you to have a drink with them; usually of some exotic Italian cordial. No matter how destitute they were, the father would always reach in somewhere and produce a dubious looking bottle. In fact there were often several bottles and father would demonstrate both his hospitality and his steadiness of hand by pouring you a pousse-café. Once a day that was a welcome lightener of the day's labors. But when you were working steadily in Italian neighborhoods, with a dozen or fifteen stops, you might as well have been a young gentleman paying New Year's calls back in Poughkeepsie. All of these first-generation immigrant families were a great relief because they never showed any surprise at having a woman doctor appear. They were used to midwives in their native lands and, after all, this was a strange and new country and there was always their innate courtesy in accepting anything they found in their new homes. They called me "doc" in all innocence of either disrespect or irony, just because an Italian cannot help cutting syllables off English words.

Towards the end of this period, it was my fate to take an active—rather too active, in fact—part in the story of Mary Mallon. Typhoid Mary, who came to have no other name, to the public at least, died on November 11, 1938, at the Riverside Hospital of the Department of Health on North Brother Island. She was seventy years old and since 1907 had been virtually a prisoner of the city. The germ of typhoid fever had been isolated in 1884 and several years later Dr. Robert Koch, a great bacteriologist, discovered during an outbreak of typhoid fever in Strassburg, Germany, that a woman who was running a bake shop in that town might be the source of the infection. She had had typhoid fever many years before and tests showed that her body still gave off the germs of typhoid. In 1904 this news came to America. Dr. George A. Soper, an eminent sanitarian, determined to find the truth of this. Starting with an epidemic of typhoid fever occurring in Mamaroneck in 1900, he had been following the trend of these numerous cases. He came upon a curious sequence of outbreaks in private families in different communities. In each family he found that the same woman was the cook, leaving shortly after the outbreak occurred to go on to her next place where, inevitably, typhoid occurred shortly afterward. She was finally located in a house on Park Avenue where several members of the family already were coming down with typhoid fever. Dr. Soper, at that time a sanitary engineer in the Department of Health, asked to have an inspector sent to get certain specimens from Mary. I was the inspector assigned to this seemingly simple task.

I learned afterward that Dr. Soper had reason to suspect that Mary might make trouble. But I knew nothing of that and, after all, I was just to get specimens of her blood and urine. When I first interviewed her, Mary was busy at her job in the kitchen of a prosperous Park Avenue household. It was the traditional brownstone-front house in the Sixties. Mary was a clean, neat, obviously self-respecting Irishwoman with a firm mouth and her hair done in a tight knot at the back of her head. Using as much routine tact as possible, I told her what I wanted. Her jaw set and her eyes glinted and she said "No." She said it in a way that left little room for persuasion or argument. Obviously here was another case of that blind, panicky distrust of doctors and all their works which crops up so often among the uneducated—and among the educated too, for that matter.

That night I received a telephone call from Dr. Bensel, my superior officer, telling me to be at the corner of Park Avenue and Sixty-seventh Street the next morning at 7:30 where I would find an ambulance and three policemen. We were to go to this house, get the blood and urine specimens and, if Mary resisted, we were to take her to the Willard Parker Hospital, by force if necessary. Of course I was there at the appointed time. Leaving the ambulance at the corner, I placed one policeman around the corner, another in front of the house and with the remaining one I went to the basement door. Mary was on the lookout and peered out, a long kitchen fork in her hand like a rapier. As she lunged at me with the fork, I stepped back, recoiled on the policeman and so confused matters that, by the time we got through the door, Mary had disappeared. "Disappear" is too matter-of-fact a word; she had completely vanished. In a three-hour search we discovered only one clue: a chair set by the high fence between this house and the adjoining one with footprints in the snow leading to it. So, much to the bewilderment of its occupants, we searched that house too; but still no Mary. The rest of the servants denied knowing anything about her or where she was; even in my distress, I liked that loyalty. Further search seemed useless. I went over to Third Avenue and telephoned Dr. Bensel that Mary could not be found. Dr. Bensel was laconic. "I expect you to get the specimens or to take Mary to the hospital." And then he rang off. On my discouraged way back to the house, I commandeered two more policemen whom I found by the way. And then we started in again. For another two hours we went through every closet and nook and cranny in those two houses. It was utter defeat. I was trying to decide how I would face Dr. Bensel, when one of the policemen caught sight of a tiny scrap of blue calico caught in the door of the areaway closet under the high outside stairway leading to the front door. A dozen filled ashcans were heaped up in front of this door; another evidence of class solidarity. The ashcans were removed and the door opened and there was Mary. Once the door was opened she wasted no time. She came out fighting and swearing, both of which she could do with appalling efficiency and vigor. I made another effort to talk to her sensibly and asked her again to let me have the specimens, but it was of no use. By that time she was convinced that the law was wantonly persecuting her, when she had done nothing wrong. She knew she had never had typhoid fever; she was maniacal in her integrity. There was nothing I could do but take her with us. The policemen lifted her into the ambulance and I literally sat on her all the way to the hospital; it was like being in a cage with an angry lion.

The hospital laboratories speedily proved that Mary was as dangerous as Dr. Soper had suspected. Her bowel movements were a living culture of typhoid bacilli. Her blood and urine showed nothing abnormal. But, as a cook, Mary could contaminate every bit of food she cooked and every dish she touched. And, to me, the interesting part of it all was that if Mary had let me have the specimens I was sent to get, she might have been a free woman all her life. It was her own bad behavior that inevitably led to her doom. The hospital authorities treated her as kindly as possible, but she never learned to listen to reason. When they suggested removing her gall-bladder, the probable focus of infection, she was convinced afresh that this was a pretext for killing her. The only answer was to keep her in the custody of the Department, out of contact with other people's food, and she was given quarters at North Brother Island in the East River.

For three years she stayed there and then was released on a solemn promise given to Dr. Ernst Lederle who was then Health Commissioner, that she would never again take any position that involved handling food. But cooking was, after all, her trade and she was constitutionally incapable of believing all this mystery about germs. So she went back to it, with the inevitable consequences. When typhoid broke out suddenly in a New Jersey sanitarium, it developed that Mary had been working there and had then run away when the disease developed. A short time later, typhoid appeared in the Sloane Maternity Hospital in New York City, with two deaths out of twenty-five cases. Although I was no longer a roving inspector, I went up there one day and walked into the kitchen. Sure enough, there was Mary earning her living in the hospital kitchen and spreading typhoid germs among mothers and babies and doctors and nurses like a destroying angel.

This time she had to go back under a life sentence, to North Brother Island. Until the other day she was still there and she still had her gall-bladder. She had threatened to kill me if she could get out, and during the years she was at large, that little doubt would stay in the back of my mind. But I could not blame her for feeling that way. From my brief acquaintance with Mary, I learned to like her and to respect her point of view. After all, she has been of great service to humanity. There have been many typhoid carriers recognized since her time but she was the first charted case and for that distinction she paid in a life-long imprisonment. Today, typhoid carriers are usually allowed their freedom, after they have pledged themselves not to handle other people's food. And, so far as we have been able to discover, they have kept their word. It was Mary's tragedy that she could not trust us.

Typhoid Mary made me realize for the first time what sweeping powers are vested in Public Health authorities. There is very little that a Board of Health cannot do in the way of interfering with personal and property rights for the protection of the public health. Boards of Health have judicial, legislative and executive powers. They are the only public agencies that combine all of these powers. It all dates back to a bad cholera epidemic in New York almost one hundred years ago, when cholera and yellow fever were still potential menaces along the Atlantic seaboard. This outbreak was so serious that a petition was sent to the State Legislature asking that emergency police measures be created for proper protection against this invasion. A Board of Health was created and, in order that it might be fully effective in any emergency, the legislature granted it extraordinary powers to use as it saw fit. These laws still persist. Today practically all Boards of Health have the same wide powers, but it is to our credit that they have used them wisely.

All of which made it strange that, in my early days, a huge municipality like New York was doing so little to control contagious diseases among children of school age. Doing anything at all was comparatively new. It was as late as the nineties that Boston and Philadelphia began pioneering in this field. I have already spoken of how pointless and sketchy school medical inspection was when I first began working for the Department. In 1902 a new administration had made an effort toward increasing the efficiency of this work, had employed additional inspectors

[77]

and begun the huge task of attempting to examine each
child periodically. The routine inspection for contagious
eye and skin diseases was done in a way that seemed farcical and yet it yielded enough information to make it worth
while. It was a rough way of finding the worst cases and
brought many of the minor ones to light. My experience
in this was the same as that of all the other medical inspectors and the same method is followed today in a large
proportion of our school systems. When I entered the room
the children all arranged themselves in a line and passed
before me in solemn procession, each child stopping for a
moment, opening his mouth hideously wide and pulling
down his lower eyelids with his fingers. For our purposes
it gave the doctor an opportunity of looking at the child's
hands (for skin diseases), his teeth, throat and eyes all at
the same time. For the children's purposes it was a beautiful opportunity for making a face at teacher unscathed
and they made the most of it. It all seems very superficial
and yet it was such a test for our quick and accurate diagnosis that we learned a great deal. After a year or two at
this sort of inspection, I reached the place where I could
pick out the undernourished children and those with other
obvious physical defects almost as soon as the door was
opened and before the children passed before me.

We started out on the principle that any case of contagious eye or skin disease must be sent home at once to
prevent the spread of any further infection. But the sheer
numbers of such cases put a stop to that scheme before
we were well started. We were literally depopulating the
schools, for the results of this first real inspection were
tragically astounding. Four out of five of these children,
about 80 per cent, had pediculosis—the polite medical term
for head-lice. One out of five, some 20 per cent, had tra-

choma, that highly infectious eye-disease which constitutes
so serious a risk of blindness that the immigration authorities no longer allow any case of it to enter the country.
You may remember that recently when they made an exception in favor of Kagawa, the Japanese people's cooperative organizer, they stipulated that a doctor would have to
stay by his side throughout his tour to guard others against
infection. The infectious skin diseases—scabies, ringworm
and impetigo—were almost as frequent. Those were not
schoolrooms we inspected; they were contagious wards with
all the different diseases so mingled it was a wonder that
each child did not have them all. Many of them did: lice,
trachoma, scabies, ringworm, all at once.

When we started sending these children home with orders to stay away from school until the infections were
well, the schoolrooms, in many schools, were practically
deserted. The children's parents were painfully astonished
at finding that Giuseppe and Isador and Sonya were being
kept out of school because of inconspicuous troubles to
which no one had ever paid any attention in the old country. That was one of our chief handicaps, of course. Our
present rigid restriction of immigration had not yet begun,
physical examination of immigrants was hardly yet exist-
ent, and the famous melting-pot of Manhattan Island had
long since become a huge germ culture. The Mediterranean
and Balkan slums and southern Russia were emptying their
underprivileged into Ellis Island and, on reaching their
new country, these underprivileged were likely to be a
definite medical and public-health problem. No one had
told them what to do about these seemingly minor ailments
and they had never known themselves that anything could
or should be done.

It was a thoroughly insane situation. Not the least ridic-

ulous detail of it appeared when the truant-officers, finding the schools emptied of pupils, began going around and
ordering these children back into school. Here was one city
department prohibiting the children from attending school
and another city department commanding the parents to
send them to school. At that point, I suppose, the children's
parents concluded that, without exception, all government
officials in this new country were crazy. It looked as though
there were no solution. The answer came as answers will
if one tries to find them. Dr. Ernst Lederle, who was then
Commissioner of Health, consulted Miss Lillian D. Wald.
Miss Wald, the well-loved and great-souled head of the
famous Henry Street Settlement, was ready to share her
knowledge of social and public-health problems with all
who might be helped. She had a solution. She would lend
the Department of Health one of her best qualified nurses,
a Miss Lina Rogers, whose common sense and wide experience might be a starting point in the right direction.
Miss Rogers turned out to be a dignified, attractive person
who exuded capability and adaptability and all of the other
required qualities. She well merits the distinction of being
the first public health nurse in this country as a result of
this task.

After Miss Rogers had carried out a few months of ex-
perimental work in a particularly bad school, we had
evolved a scheme to check these minor infections. Our war
on pediculosis in the New York City slums (aided by the
restriction of immigration), for instance, has turned a mat-
ter-of-course condition into a disgrace. The method of
attack was home-missionary work, teaching whole families
that a shampoo and fine-tooth comb technique followed
by soaking the hair in kerosene to kill the nits would accomplish our purpose. I can still see the lines of little girls

with their pigtails pulled forward over their eyes so that
the nurse could look through their hair. There were hazards about this job. All nurses periodically acquired lice
themselves. Even I, who seldom had to do that work of
inspection, have not avoided that infection on several occasions.

For the care of the infectious skin diseases, we planned
a readily applied protective treatment to keep the infection
from spreading. When treated, the children could stay
safely in school without danger of spreading the infection
to others. We established a clinic in each school, supplied
with simple remedies, and the children reported each day
to the nurse for the appropriate treatment. We could not
take any chance with trachoma; it was too serious a disease.
So we solved that problem in a different way. Throughout
the city we established special classes in the schools for
these affected children. They could go on with their studies
but were not allowed any contact with the other children
in the schools. For the worst cases, we had special clinics
where children who could not be allowed in school could
have the specialized treatment necessary, or where operations that had to be done could be performed with safety
and skill. These clinics were crowded for many years but
were given up long ago as trachoma has now sunk to the
vanishing point. That was another victory.

As a result of Miss Rogers' experiments, the Department
installed her technique in other schools and employed several more nurses to carry it out. Eventually the school
nurse with her equipment and medicines and shrewd willingness to go as far as was advisable without a doctor's
advice was known all over the city. Today, there is hardly
a place in the United States that does not support a school
nurse. The results were quite as astonishing to me as the

appalling conditions the nurses were combatting. How much school nurses have accomplished was vividly brought home to me a few years ago when I was teaching a course in public health at Teachers College, Columbia University, and made a practice of taking my students down to a public school for a first-hand lesson in the technique of inspecting school children. Naturally I wanted plenty of cases of contagious eye and skin diseases for demonstration, so I asked the Superintendent of Nurses to have sent to me every available case of pediculosis, scabies, trachoma, ringworm and impetigo to be found in the Borough of Manhattan. The response was breathtaking—because it was so meager. In all of the Borough of Manhattan they could never produce more than two or three cases of any given infection, whereas fifteen years before we had had them by the hundreds in every public school. Our care and treatment had been an overwhelming success—a magnificent tribute to the splendid and thorough work of the school nursing staff.

By this time my attitude toward public health problems was approaching a definite plan. I did not yet know the exact answer I expected, but I had a feeling that it was just around the corner. It was. That corner was turned when I was assigned to work with a group from the Bureau of Municipal Research—a privately financed organization which was always looking into and checking up on details of city affairs where political administrations were too ignorant, too cautious or too lazy to bother to seek out the facts. At that time the Bureau was managed by Henry Bruere, now president of the great Bowery Savings Bank, William H. Allen, a well known investigator, and Paul Wilson, husband of Frances Perkins, the present Secretary of Labor—keen people, all of them. When they started investigating New York City's scandalous death rate, I was assigned to cooperate with them as politely as possible.

It might have been just another assignment. But in the course of their study, the Bureau turned up one set of facts that made me stop, look and listen. Of all the people who died in New York City every year, a third were children under five years of age and a fifth were babies less than a year old. It was the babies and small children who never really had a chance to live, who swelled the death rate to fantastically macabre proportions. Interesting figures beyond any doubt; perhaps they impressed me so particularly because they were not just cold statistics to me at all. I had served my time in that long, hot summer in Hell's Kitchen when I walked up and down tenement stairs to find in every house a wailing skeleton of a baby, doomed by ignorance and neglect to die needlessly. I had interviewed mother after mother too ignorant to know that precautions could be taken and too discouraged to bother taking them even when you tried to teach her. If mothers could be taught what to do, most of these squalid tragedies need never happen. The way to keep people from dying from disease, it struck me suddenly, was to keep them from falling ill. Healthy people didn't die. That sounds like a completely absurd and witless remark, but at that time it really was a startling idea; at any rate it seemed so to me. And I found that it was when I tried to convince the authorities that something might be done about teaching people how to stay well.

Preventive medicine had hardly been born yet and had no portion in public-health work. People were speaking of Colonel Gorgas' work in cleaning tropical diseases out of the Canal Zone as if he had been a mediaeval archangel performing miracles with a flaming sword instead of a brilliant apostle of common sense and sound information in combatting epidemics. The great campaign to prevent and combat tuberculosis with Dr. Herman M. Biggs as its fine leader was still in its infancy. At that time health departments went entirely on the principle that there was no point in doing much until something had happened. If a person fell ill with a contagious disease, you quarantined him; if he committed a nuisance you made him stop doing it or made him pay the penalty. It was all after-the-fact effort—locking the stable door after the horse was stolen; pretty hopeless in terms of permanent results. No, there was no preventive medicine in public health. The term "Public Health Education" had not been invented. Perhaps something might be done; I was not sure but I hoped it could be tried.

The Bureau of Municipal Research group and I saw this at the same time. They had authority; I had none. And then they recommended to the Department that a division should be established to deal with the matter. Dr. Darlington and Dr. Bensel were favorable to the idea. Dr. Bensel called me into his office one day in the early summer of 1908 to tell me I might have a try at it. I came out of that office the proud and bewildered Chief of the newly created Division of Child Hygiene. I had no staff; I had no money; all I had was an idea. It was clear to the Commissioner that it was going to be a struggle to convince the Board of Estimate and Apportionment that money could be legally appropriated to care for well people. I could see that myself. A large part of being a successful government administrator consists of being able to keep the political powers-that-be appropriating funds for your pet projects; that is as true today as it always has been. You have to be a salesman as well as an executive. As a salesman I was going to need an impressive sample before I could get into our budget a sum large enough to pay for any such experiment. It had to be more than an idea: it must be something concrete and definite if the money was to be forthcoming.

After several consultations as to how this approach might be made, I was allowed a trial experiment. The closing of schools in June would mean that the thirty-odd nurses on school inspection duty would be at liberty. June also meant the beginning of the diarrhoeal season which, if this summer of 1908 was going to be anything like its predecessors, would kill its 1500 babies each week all through the hot weather. The Commissioner and Dr. Bensel let me have those nurses to use in an experiment in preventive child hygiene.

In order to make our experiment count for something, the scheme had to be tried out first in a district with a very high baby death rate. So I selected a complicated, filthy, sunless and stifling nest of tenements on the lower east side of the city. If we could accomplish anything in the face of living conditions like these, we would go far toward proving our point. This neighborhood was largely populated by recently landed Italians, willing to learn new things in a new country. Mrs. Capozzi might be puzzled to find a perfect stranger dropping in to tell her how to take care of her perfectly well baby, but there was probably as much point in learning the American way of caring for babies as there was in learning the American way of talking.

How to reach the newborn babies without any waste effort was a problem. But it was not too difficult to solve. The Registrar of Records in the Department was cooperative and used to each day send me the name and address

on the birth certificate of every baby whose birth had been
reported on the previous day. It was essential to reach these
babies while they were still very young and this proved
to be the ideal way to find them; it is still the ideal way.
Within a few hours, a graduate nurse, thoroughly instructed in the way to keep a well baby well, visited the
address to get acquainted with the mother and her baby
and go into the last fine detail of just how that baby should
be cared for. Nothing revolutionary; just insistence on
breast-feeding, efficient ventilation, frequent bathing, the
right kind of thin summer clothes, out-of-door airing in the
little strip of park around the corner—all of it commonplace enough for the modern baby, but all of it completely
new to Mrs. Capozzi and all of it new in public health.
Many of these mothers were a little flattered to have an
American lady take all that trouble about little Giovanni,
and were likely to go out of their way to learn and to cooperate. If the mothers were sulky or apprehensive, the
nurses went again and again, wearing down their resistance, establishing friendly contact, until they were ready
and willing to cooperate. In my experience, nearly all
mothers are fine when they are given half a chance to
know how to be. As soon as they saw that their babies were
flourishing, despite the cruelly hot weather, they became
our most efficient aides.

From the first I was pretty sure that we were getting
results. I was not prepared, however, for the impressiveness
of the facts when the results of the summer's campaign
in that corner of the east side were tabulated. During that
summer there were 1200 fewer deaths in that district than
there had been the previous summer; we had saved more
babies than there were men in a regiment of soldiers and
I had learned one certain thing: heat did not necessarily

kill babies. Everywhere else in town the summer death rate of babies had been quite as bad as ever. We had found out how to save babies on a large scale. But it was far more important that we had proved that prevention paid far beyond our wildest hopes. There, if we have to be dramatic about it, was the actual beginning of my life work.

Early in August the Department officially created the Division of Child Hygiene with me as its Chief. Money came from the Board of Estimate and Apportionment in fairly generous amounts. It did very nicely as a beginning. Before I left the Department, however, our annual appropriation was well over twelve hundred thousand dollars a year. The first Bureau of Child Hygiene in the world was on its way.

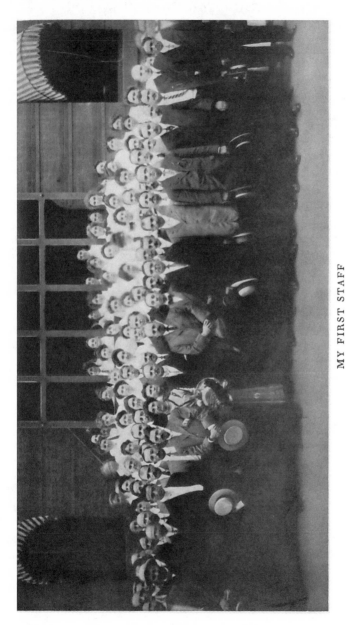

MY FIRST STAFF

The doctors and nurses of the Bureau of Child Hygiene in 1909

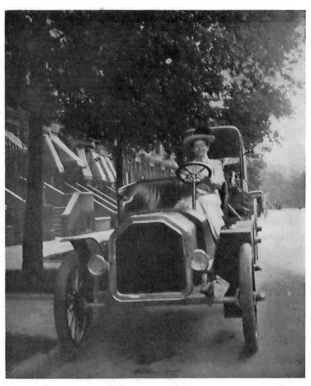

STARTING OUT FOR A DAY'S WORK, *CIRCA* 1912

CHAPTER V

IT WAS NEVER QUITE CLEAR IN MY MIND
whether in pioneering in child hygiene being a woman was
more of an asset than a liability. There were many times
when a man might bury himself under the anonymity of
his sex in such a position and thus contrive to get many
things done without comment or criticism. But for a
woman, this was more difficult. There were many stumbling
blocks and the first one came early. It is difficult to realize
now, but at that time the appointment of a woman as an
executive was an upturning of procedure that brought out
trouble all along the way. On the other hand, it had its
compensations. From the point of view of publicity, it was
superb. I have a well-defined feeling that if a man had been
given this position, it would have been just another bureau;
but for a woman to get this job, well, that was news. The
Bureau needed publicity; my sex offered a challenge that
provided good copy for the reporters and one of my real
problems was how to avoid publicity instead of seeking it.
That challenge was met immediately.

The start came when I was assigned a staff. Naturally
they were all men. I had previously worked with all of
them; we were good friends in our lowly capacity of inspectors. The picked few who were to help me form the
Bureau were doctors; all splendid men, able, conscientious
and adjustable. But evidently not adjustable enough to take
kindly to the idea of working for a woman. They had

hardly received notice of their appointments when all six
of them walked solemnly into my office and told me that
they had submitted their resignations. It was nothing personal, they assured me, but they could not reconcile themselves to the idea of taking orders from a woman. This was
an impasse that I had not thought about but it was a serious
one. I had to think quickly. I needed those particular doctors; I wanted them to work with me. It was a rather tense
moment and I asked them to sit down and talk it over with
me. "See here," I said; "you are really crying before you
are hurt. I quite realize that you may not like the idea of
working under me as a woman. But isn't there another side
of this question? I do not know whether I am going to like
working with you. None of us know how this is going to
turn out. But if I am willing to take the responsibilty of
our success or failure, I think you might take a sporting
chance with me."

They looked thoughtful for a long moment but no one
said anything. I had to go on. "Let's try it this way. Give
the arrangement a month's trial. If at the end of a month
you still do not like it, go ahead and resign, and I will not
say anything about it. But, if all goes well and you want
to stay, I shall be glad. Is that agreed?"

They pondered again for a few moments and then, not
too enthusiastically, said they would stay and hold up their
resignations for a month. That month went by and I reminded them that the time had come for their decision.
All of them told me that they had withdrawn their resignations. They had completely recovered from their dis-
tressful doubts and sensibilities. By that time we were all
in the midst of an interesting and enthralling job and, as I
had hoped, they were much too keen about its possibilities
to leave it for a moment. Besides, with what now seems

almost like Machiavellian subtlety, I had given each one a
title and placed him at the head of a division in the Bureau.
All six of those men stayed with me during the critical
years of organization. Dr. John J. Cronin, Dr. Royall
Willis, Dr. Jacob Sobel and Dr. Robert Fowler were with
the Bureau until I retired. Dr. William Weber died in
harness as chief of the baby health stations. Dr. Clarence
Smith eventually retired to look after his thriving practice,
but not until the spadework of experiment and organization
was finished. I owe a tremendous debt of gratitude to all
of them. They were at my right hand for many years and
no one could have had a more loyal, a more efficient or a
finer set of co-workers. For Superintendent of Nurses, I
had Miss Anna Kerr, an able and effective administrator.
They were all splendid friends.

There were other places where being a woman was useful. In politics, for instance. I still knew no more about
politics than I had learned from the famous Job Hedges,
the celebrated wit and after-dinner speaker. I met him one
day when he was running for the office of Governor of
New York State. I knew him very well from the old days
when he was a very young man and I was a little girl in
Dansville, so I asked him if he thought he was going to
be elected. "No, I can't be elected," he said. "People think
I am a funny man. And the first rule of politics is that, if
you are funny, you can be popular and you will be laughed
at but you cannot be elected because no one will ever take
you seriously." He was right. He was not elected and I
think that was the reason. Anyway, I did not forget that
piece of advice and it was many years before I dared tell
a funny story before an audience. But I was still anything
but a professional politician. I had gone into the Department of Health solely because it promised to pay a salary

for very little work and I spent my entire career there fighting shy of politics.

But the Department was part of the political set-up of a politics-ridden big city and on many and many an occasion not even an apprehensive innocent like myself could avoid becoming a part of this game. When as head of this new Bureau I was endowed with the right to suggest or influence appointments, the trouble began and never stopped until I retired. And here, being a woman was an enlightening asset in dealing with the old-time Tammany crew of chieftains and hangers-on. No one has ever been quite able to define Tammany Hall in its old days; indeed it would present its difficulties today. They well knew how to make men knuckle down and obey orders, but they had no previous experience of women in a political office. Between their bewilderment over that anomaly and their natural Irish politeness, I could often find my right way out. What is more, I came to like the Tammany groups that I met. I liked them and I liked to work with them. That is heresy, I know, but I couldn't help it. There was "The" McManus, a quiet and gentlemanly sort when I saw him, whatever he may have been on the outside. "Big Tim" Sullivan was another man who always was courteous and charming to me, and Senator Pat McCarren who had the richest brogue of them all and the greatest sense of what was due to "a lady." There were many more but these are the men who stand out in my memory. I was not innocent enough not to know their background. Fundamentally, I was opposed to Tammany and all it stood for. But given an individual contact with its leading lights, I learned to know the game and could still like the men who played it.

They had a curious honesty in their approach. They knew what they wanted and asked for it. But, because I

was a woman, they were very polite about it and the effect
was that they were asking a favor of me instead of giving
me orders. They were always sending me incredible women
to be appointed as nurses; this had happened many times
when I was still assistant to the Commissioner. Our nurses
were not under civil service at first, so candidates had no
examination to pass and, theoretically, we could appoint
anyone who had the wit to say she was a nurse, whether or
not she had ever seen so much as the entrance door to a
hospital. Up to a point, I had played ball with Tammany
in the interests of a quiet life. In the very early days, if
the woman was fit for children to be with and had had any
reasonable experience, she was appointed. But in those days,
many of them were not only distinctly not nurses but, having become the cast-off sweethearts of Tammany ward-
heelers, were not to be endowed with city jobs. One day
Senator McCarren sent me a fine specimen of that type,
who had, no doubt, started life in a sailors' dance hall on
the Brooklyn waterfront. I listened to her for two minutes,
asked her to step outside, and then got the Senator on the
telephone.

"I'm sorry," I told him, "but it just can't be done. You
know as well as I do that this woman is not the sort of
person who should associate with children."

"You mean," he said, "you don't think the lady and
children would mix?"

"I do not," I said, "and what is more, she isn't a nurse.
I am not even sure she knows what the word means."

"Well," he said, "no doubt you're right. I haven't seen
her myself. I'll just tell Senator Blank his girl will have to
get a job somewheres else." Then I heard him chuckle at
the other end of the wire. "Ye're a true lady," he said,

"and I like to see such a broth of a girl standing up to Tammany. I'll stand by you, doctor."

The fact that the politicians and I mutually liked one another helped a great deal, of course. At bottom they were thoroughly corrupt and cynical, a sort of government cancer, but my occasional half-hour chats with these bosses were almost invariably very pleasant occasions. They all seemed to like me, all except the great McCooey of Brooklyn. He and I fell out because, when he called me up and ordered me to send him the list of nurses who had then passed the civil service examinations so he could tell me which ones were to be appointed, I refused. By that time the whole matter of the nursing staff had been settled by making them civil service employees. Their appointment was covered by the civil service rules, for which I was profoundly grateful. I had no desire, nor in fact any authority, to pass this over to any politician, no matter how great he might be. But from that time on, I faced almost overwhelming resistance to anything I wanted to do in his kingdom of Brooklyn. His power was very great there and woe betide anyone who dared oppose him.

Sometimes I went to Tammany for the help I could not get from the city government. We would often find a baby in a family completely on the ragged edge, starving and freezing. Organized charity acted too slowly in such cases. So here was the cue for dropping in on the local Tammany district leader, who kept up his political fences by handing out help wherever it was needed. Two minutes of description, then: "Sure, ma'am, he'll get a sack of coal and enough money to eat on right away." Naturally the family so assisted meant another vote for the Tammany candidate in the next election, but that was not my business in such an emergency. If the head of the family played his cards right, Tammany would probably see that he got a job. All of which does count on the credit side for Tammany.

To be quite honest, I must confess that I would rather work with a Tammany administration than with a reform administration. I know, and knew then, that the organization meant graft and wholesale corruption. In the shameful conditions in the Health Department in my early days I had seen at close range where that sort of thing led. But, as the head of a Bureau trying to get things done, I inevitably had to depend upon the administration in power, and Tammany's methods, in my case, were a comfort. When I took a new idea to a reform administration, they were always very gentlemanly about it. But it was a long and arduous road to follow. They would, of course, ask how much it would cost and then, after they had studied my carefully worked out statement which went into meticulous detail, they would send me word that it would be considered in due course. Months later, they would let me know that although the idea was fundamentally sound, the state of the city's finances made it inadvisable at the moment. I did not want things considered; I wanted them done. Their caution appeared to be in the taxpayers' interest, of course, but from my point of view it was not the way to get things accomplished, and in the long run the taxpayers were bound to suffer too. I knew my work was important and I knew that it would always be an up-hill fight to put it over. It would have been far the easier way to rest upon these vague promises and sink back into inertia. There were brilliant exceptions, of course. George McAneny, who was at one time President of the Board of Aldermen, and Paul Wilson, who was secretary to Mayor John Purroy Mitchel, were men of social vision and gave me great help as well as moral support, but on the whole reform administrations were hard sledding for reformers.

When a Tammany administration was in power there was no such hanging fire. The Mayor and other heads at City Hall were too exalted and busy to be approached directly but there was always another and less direct route to follow. Always an eminent Tammanyite who could be approached and told what was on my mind and how great the need was. He rarely asked questions; just, "So you're sure it's a good idea, Doctor. But then it's always a good idea to help the babies;" and when I had said yes, he would say, "And why not? I'll let the right people know and you'll get your appropriation." And that was that. In ways that might be devious, the plan I wanted to follow would be financed in the next budget for the Health Department. There was never any question of a *quid pro quo*. And this baffling mixture of official incompetence explained to me, in part at least, Tammany's hold on the people: large spending and innate humanity. Incidentally, it is interesting to look back today upon the "wild orgy of spending" of the Tammany regimes, and reflect upon the mounting budgets of the present.

I took only one piece of graft while I worked for the Department. I still have it somewhere. One morning while I was assistant to Dr. Darlington, the Department doorman came in and said there was a man outside who had a present for me. With the Department's shy evasion of the woman question, I was then officially "Dr. S. J. Baker," on the letterheads at least. The man said he was a barber. I did not want any presents from barbers or from anyone else and told the doorman to send him away. In ten minutes he returned, saying the man had left but that he had insisted on leaving the present as his "thank you" for a

letter I had written him. I opened it out of curiosity and
found a gorgeous shaving mug tastefully inscribed "Dr.
S. J. Baker" in large gold letters. It was the kind of shaving mug that barber shops used to present to steady patrons
and keep in special shelves by the mirror. I have another
which belonged to my father; they make a noble pair. I
could not resist keeping it.

I had few opportunities to be tempted. Only once in a
very long while some woman looking for a permit to board
a baby would try to buy herself what she wanted. To their
credit, I know of no midwife who ever tried to buy her
permit. And we had nothing else to sell. So graft did not
rear its ugly head in the Bureau of Child Hygiene. But,
throughout the Department, it would come out into the
open often enough. There was the periodic scandal in a
few of the Bureaus at regular intervals; generally at the
beginning of each new administration. It was usually concerned with food: just a quiet slipping the inspector a hundred dollar bill and suggesting that he might prefer to
look at this car of vegetables instead of the shipment four
cars down the line. A certain number of inspectors were
dismissed and sometimes a jail sentence waited for them
but after the cleaning-up was over and everything quiet
again, the same graft crept in once more. The same conditions occurred in the milk division at one time and that
resulted in sending a highly placed official of the Department to Sing Sing prison for a five-year sentence. Later,
one of the most important officials in the Department decided to clean up this situation for good and all. He did it
too but when things became too warm to be pleasant, he
was offered a large salary to resign and go over to a certain
large milk concern to reorganize that business so that such

conditions could not occur any longer. He went, and was left in solitary grandeur in an office of his own until after a year or two he found himself out of a job. But the purpose had been accomplished; he had been taken out of the Department. Whether such conditions hold now, I do not know. I can only speak of my time.

Disgusting, of course. But that is politics. No doubt that story made such an impression on me because when I heard it I had also had a long time of being under fire. It is, to me, a remarkable story and ties me up with no less a person than Mayor John F. Hylan, "Red Mike" himself.

Mr. Hylan came into office as mayor in 1918 as a reaction to John Purroy Mitchel's famous reform administration. Previous to his election I had never seen the man in my life. After a chance to study him at close range, I agreed with the newspaper editorial which commented about him that "if his ability had been equal to his courage, he would have been a great mayor." A huge, handsome, red-haired giant whom I was prepared to like, even though there was little possibility that he would ever mean anything more to me than a shadowy figure down at City Hall who would, like all other mayors, always be in the papers for one reason or another. As Commissioner of Health, Mr. Hylan appointed Dr. J. Lewis Amster, a highly respected, honest and capable physician from the Bronx. That sounded fine. But the day after Dr. Amster took office, I found that Mayor Hylan was going to mean a great deal to me during the next years. The Commissioner sent for me, shook my hand and then, almost blushing:

"I don't know what this is all about," he said, "but I have strict instructions from the Mayor to dismiss you at once."

I had to make him repeat it before I could grasp what he had said. Then I asked why on earth the Mayor should want me dismissed.

"I don't know," said Dr. Amster. "There's no explanation, just an order to get you out of the Department at once."

The man was so patently telling the truth, so obviously just as bewildered as I, that I had to accept the situation and fight.

"But you can't dismiss me just like that," I said. "I'm under civil service. You'll have to investigate my conduct in office and prefer charges against me."

There was nothing for Dr. Amster to do but report my defiance to those higher up. They instructed him to keep right on with the battle to throw me out by hook or crook. The poor man evidently bothered his superiors a good deal about it—until at last he secured for me a vague inkling of what it was all about.

"The Mayor says," he told me, "that you once worked for the Rockefellers and that you are still in their pay and he will not stand for having a capitalist spy in his administration." (It must be remembered that Mayor Hylan was not a Tammany figure—he was backed by Tammany in the election, but primarily he was the candidate of William Randolph Hearst who was going in at a great rate for muckraking the interests at that time.) Dr. Amster was quite pleased, as he might well have been, to have turned up a plausible reason for the way the Mayor was hunting my scalp—he thought it made a kind of sense out of a lunatic situation. I hated to disappoint a nice man, but, on this basis, the thing made less sense than ever, as I told him. I had never worked for the Rockefellers—the only payroll I had ever been on was the city's.

We parted, each more bewildered than ever. Presently, as the prodding from higher up grew more and more pronounced, Dr. Amster could stand it no longer. He called me in again and said:

"I'm going to resign. And it is mainly on your account. I've asked about you in all directions and everybody says you're all right. You may have some enemies, but I can't find them. And by this time I don't see why I should look any farther, no matter what the Mayor wants. So," he said, holding out his hand, "I'm out. Good luck to you."

I shook that hand very heartily indeed. It was a really fine gesture. To have been Commissioner of Health, with all the prestige and power that position carried, and then drop it because you were asked unreasonably to persecute an under-official whom you had never known before—that was real integrity.

In appointing the next Commissioner Mr. Hylan outdid himself in his own peculiar way. The story was that he met on the street a man he knew who was accompanied by the late Dr. Royal S. Copeland, then an eye-specialist with nothing whatever to do with politics. The friend introduced Dr. Copeland to the Mayor—the Mayor took one look at him and said: "I like your looks, Doctor. The Commissioner of Health has just resigned—how would you like the job?" Dr. Copeland made the obvious answer that he knew a good deal about astigmatism and cataracts but nothing whatever about public health work. "What of it?" said Mr. Hylan. "You're a doctor, aren't you? Think it over— the job's yours if you want it." Dr. Copeland thought it over, telephoned the Mayor the next day that he would like the job if it were still open—and so started on a political career that finally landed him in the United States Senate with a well-deserved reputation as the biggest vote-getter in New York State. That was the one constructive result of the Mayor's unrelenting efforts to eject me from my well fortified position.

Within a few days Dr. Copeland took over the Commissioner's post and the game of "Get Dr. Baker" was resumed along exactly the same lines, again with the Mayor insisting that I was a Rockefeller spy and nobody else able to understand the situation at all. By this time Mr. Hylan had added the detail that I was a product of the Mitchel administration, which he loathed, and that was another good reason for getting rid of me. I explained at length to Dr. Copeland that I knew none of the Rockefellers, had never seen a cent of their money, and had originally been appointed, not by Mayor Mitchel but in 1901 when R. A. Van Wyck was Mayor. I convinced Dr. Copeland but neither he nor anyone else could convince the Mayor that he was wrong. Then the Mayor took the battle into his own hands and, for over two years, my time was wasted, my disposition frayed and the Bureau's work demoralized by this unwarranted persecution.

The Mayor filled my office with investigators, combing through the files, asking everybody questions, looking mysterious and getting sadly in the way. They found nothing. He went around and asked about me from all the big medical societies, state and county—and, prod as he might, they gave me a clean bill of health. It was all done quietly, but the newspapers got wind of it and there began to appear hints that, if the Bureau of Child Hygiene, which was by all odds the most popular activity of the whole Department, was not let alone, trouble would commence. The Commissioner of Accounts' office gave me a thorough going-over. I was called up before ex-Judge David Hirshfield in private and semi-private hearings in which he went far out of his way to be unpleasant. Then the Civil Service Commission took me in hand using gentler but equally fruitless methods. Then they passed me over to the City Chamberlain for more weeks of defensive warfare. And all the while the office was full of investigators so it was impossible to get my work done even when I had time and energy. They finally got into such a state of frustrated bewilderment that they could only grunt when I would offer to help them if they would only tell me what they were looking for.

"Just give me a lead," I would say when a new one appeared, "and maybe I can turn up something for you. I'll be glad to help—this is boring me to death and I want it over with." They had an unhappy time, poor souls, forced by reasons that never existed to go on looking for something that wasn't there.

Fortunately this was in 1919, when the Bureau was pretty well organized along its main lines, so it could stand the strain of demoralization and curtailed appropriations and all varieties of political sabotage without going absolutely to pieces. And it was heartening to see how the press and private organizations rallied to my aid as word spread that I was under fire. There were impassioned editorials and front-page stories warning the Mayor that public opinion would not stand for interference with my work in the Bureau. Things like this, to quote from the New York *Globe* and thereby blow my own horn a little: "The main reason that more than nine hundred in every thousand of our babies survive their first year is that a woman of rare intelligence looks after them. Dr. Josephine Baker for many years has done a bit of work that has meant a great deal to the city and to the nation, as well as to educate every man and woman in the duties and privileges of existence." The county medical societies and the New York Academy of Medicine, with whom I had so often crossed swords in the past, passed resolutions of unqualified endorsement for my work. So did many private welfare societies—there was hardly a day when the papers did not have some such red-hot shot to fire across the Mayor's bows. Individuals of all kinds came to see me to offer help and finally a group of mothers whose babies had been cared for by the Bureau marched in a group to the Mayor's office to protest against his incomprehensible behavior. It all added up to irresistible pressure, and after weary months of this bad dream, the Mayor relaxed his efforts and I started picking up the pieces at the Bureau.

The explanation came presently. One day Dr. Copeland telephoned me, saying that the Mayor wanted some pictures of himself holding a baby—election time was coming near, I think—and wouldn't I arrange a collection of babies at one of our baby health stations? I went there myself at the appointed hour to make sure things went smoothly. The Mayor came in with Dr. Copeland and Dr. Copeland presented me nervously: "Mr. Mayor, this is Dr. Baker, the head of the Bureau of Child Hygiene."

The Mayor shook hands unenthusiastically, saying:

"How do you do, Dr. Davis?"

Things began vaguely to dawn on me:

"I'm not Dr. Davis," I said; "I'm Dr. Baker—Dr. Josephine Baker."

He gave me a puzzled glance and looked away.

"It's all right, Dr. Davis," he said and picked up a baby.

I gave Dr. Copeland one look and rushed into the back room where I could laugh by myself. When I spoke of my theory to Dr. Copeland, who knew the Mayor far better than I did, he agreed with me absolutely. All of this time the Mayor had been persecuting me under the delusion that I was somebody else—Dr. Katharine Bement Davis, who really *had* been appointed Commissioner of Corrections by Mayor Mitchel, *had* been employed by the Rockefeller Foundation. I suppose that, since she had had the bad luck to be the only woman in a public job who had ever penetrated Mr. Hylan's consciousness, it followed that, whatever anybody said, or my birth-certificate certified, I, as a woman in a public job, would always be Katharine Bement Davis so far as he was concerned. It still gives me an uncanny feeling to think of it. Skeptical readers may disbelieve that story if they wish, but it is unqualifiedly true.

A minor—extremely minor—consolation for all the trouble caused by Mr. Hylan's insistence that I was somebody else consisted of the huge amount of publicity the Bureau received—column after column of it, all heartwarmingly laudatory and highly useful. I had to be something of a press agent in this job, because the more the newspapers mentioned the Bureau, the better luck we would have with the politicians in getting funds and cooperation. Publicity was our best defense against budget-cutting and inter-departmental sniping, and, as a natural result of our willingness to oblige, reporters came to count on us for copy. And babies are good copy, Heaven bless them. The emphasis, of course, was always on the Bureau, its work with mothers and children, its achievements and ambition. But the fact that there was a woman-executive at the head of it apparently making good and blazing trails where men had never bothered to explore was a fine angle and did no harm at all.

I was trying to maintain a paradoxical position. On the one hand, in the Department itself, I tried to make every-

one forget that I was a woman. Outside, and for the purpose of making the Bureau well and widely known, it
seemed to me fair game to get all the publicity possible.
The woman angle was still "news" and reporters were almost daily visitors at my office. Once, the combination of
a very hot afternoon, a harassed reporter and a story-
hungry editor put me personally on the front page of
almost every newspaper in the country and left me in the
position of wishing I could run away to Patagonia to escape
the headlines. On a dull and super-hot day in midsummer,
this particular reporter wandered into my office and told
me he simply had to have a story. Nothing of any importance was happening in the world and any story, no matter how unimportant, could be used. I had no ideas and
neither had he; it was that kind of a day. Finally my eye
fell upon a little leaflet which we had just printed containing advice to mothers about hot-weather care of the baby.
This included, most inconspicuously, an item to the effect
that the fewer clothes a baby wore during the hot weather
the better off he would be; in fact that it was a good idea
to take all his clothes off and let him play indoors on a
sheet on the floor during the hottest part of the day. Every
modern mother knows and does this, but it was a startling
idea then. My reporter went away with his leaflet, pretty
disconsolate. I do not know what story he turned in but I
do know what the editor made of it and in that day and
age it was considered sufficiently startling to be sent to as
many other papers as possible.

The next morning that particular reporter's paper and
all of the other morning papers blossomed out with front
page stories headed "Back to Eve," "September Morn" or
equally intriguing titles. The story said that I recommended that all babies should go naked all summer and the

idea was played up from every possible angle. Now that nudism has accustomed the public to all such ideas that story would not be worth printing. This, however, was many years ago, and it went all over the country like wildfire. All summer the newspapers played wilder and wilder changes on Dr. Baker's recommendation of nakedness instead of straw hats and lemonade. At the end, they were running what, no doubt, were very daring cartoons for that day, of respectable gentlemen wearing only the most abbreviated shorts, walking down Fifth Avenue cool and cheerful with umbrellas between them and a blazing sun. It became known as the "September Morn" theory, produced elaborate humorous prophecies of the ruin of the cotton industry, was dinned into my ears until I was as frantic on the subject as ever Anthony Comstock was when he had the art-gallery prosecuted for displaying the famous picture in its window. I had never realized before how much an ingenious newspaperman could make out of how little when he had to.

In fact I seemed to be haunted by the fantastic and bizarre in those early years. There was the nurse, new to the Bureau, who eventually called herself to the attention of her superiors by her curious habit of taking leave of absence on both Christian and Jewish holidays. That is more or less routine in the New York business office, but in our work, where a skeleton staff had to be kept on, holidays or not, it was a matter for some comment. So I called her in, the next time she applied for a holiday, whether Yom Kippur or Easter I do not remember, and asked:

"This is just a natural piece of inquiry, Miss So-and-so. You have been applying for both Christian and Jewish holidays. Just what is your religion?"

"My religion?" she said. "Well, people always think it's

a little funny in a nurse. I'm a Christian Scientist, Doctor."

Personally, besides, I have occasionally got into remarkably bizarre situations due entirely to the fact that my father was named Baker and my middle name, which I used customarily, was Josephine. It was all right until after the war, when that sensational colored stage-dancer, whose name also happened to be Josephine Baker, became the sensation of Paris and all Europe. If I had been aware that a namesake of mine had become the reigning toast of the Paris music-halls the same summer I was planning to go abroad, I might have had my passport issued to "Sara J. Baker." But I had no idea. And the consequence was that my summer in Europe was the quintessence of absurdity.

It was bad enough in Paris, where that name in the hotel list of the Paris *Herald* brought flocks of the lady's would-be admirers crowding into the lobby to stare at me and go away mystified. My room-telephone was besieged by all the milliners and dressmakers in Paris, insisting that Mademoiselle Baker always let them come to show her things and purchased very liberally. My increasingly frantic refusals to have anything to do with them probably gave the whole world of Parisian couturières the impression that Josephine Bay-ker-r-r-r had fallen on hard times. And then, when I left Paris for a couple of months' traveling through Italy and Central Europe, I had the bad luck to choose a route about two weeks ahead of a tour which my *alter ego* was making. I got her mail in Palermo, Naples and Rome. In Vienna and Budapest I didn't dare leave my right name when ordering something at a shop because, when I would return for a fitting, I always found a mob surrounding the store, waiting for a glimpse of the famous dancer. The climax came in Brussels. When I asked for my mail at my hotel there, the concierge said there was none.

I was expecting an important letter at that address, so I insisted that he look again, and repeated my name as loudly and clearly and Frenchifiedly as I could. That brought the manager out of an inner office—he looked at me, blinked and asked my name again. I showed my passport to prove it. You never saw a man so crestfallen. But he did reach up into a special cubbyhole and produced my letter.

"Ah, madame," he said, "I put it there with my own hands so none but myself would have the honor of presenting it to the renommée Josephine Bay-kère-r-r-r—" And he almost wept as he gave it to me.

A few seasons ago I went to see my namesake performing on the New York stage. I can see why he was so cut up about it.

CHAPTER VI

ALL THIS GOSSIPING, HOWEVER, HAS KEPT ME away from the story of the Bureau itself, which is, after all, the main point. Once I was in that job, I stayed in it till I retired. This is a one-track story.

Fortunately for me, my checkered past of playing factotum for the Department of Health had long since cured me of any apprehension about striking out in a new job. I did not appeal to myself as a pioneer in a new field, however—there was nothing so rhetorical about it as that. It was just that here was something that needed doing and should be approached in the most practical way. If someone had come up to us and said, with a light in his eye: "Ladies and gentlemen, you are doing a great humanitarian task that has never been done before!" we would only have said: "Not really?" and gone on figuring out whether or not that vacant delicatessen store on Avenue A would do for a new baby health station. We did not have time to dramatize ourselves.

Nevertheless, little as we realized it, we had a tremendous technical and strategical advantage in the fact that we were pioneering. There were no precedents to hamper us, no body of established knowledge to prevent us from seeing needs and remedies clearly and directly. Our one guiding principle was to start babies healthy and keep them so and, if that objective led us into far fields, all the way from the young east-side bride's diet to the habits of certain herds of cows in Jersey, we could go right along without wondering if our procedure were orthodox. As I look back, I can even be glad that we started with relatively little money and that our budget-increases, which eventually made us the most expensive bureau in the Department, came with tantalizing slowness. With neither time nor money to waste, we had to cut clean to the bone and eliminate waste motion as religiously as if it had been the eighth deadly sin.

Even in a little detail like records we had to cut our coat according to our cloth and were all the better for it. When the Bureau first started, it was endowed with a set of records specially worked out for it by the Bureau of Municipal Research. This was a fine institution but it knew very little about children and had a fetish about record keeping. The cards they gave us for school inspection required inspector and clerk to fill out the same form with the same information *eleven* times. I had visions of my whole meager staff with heads bowed down over clerical work and no time for anything else. The nurses' cards were just as bad. Night after night I labored over drawing up a set of forms to simplify matters and yet get all useful information into the indicated hands—and then one happy day I threw out the old lot and put my new forms into operation. It was like cleaning sand out of the gear-box of a car. To this day around seventy-five percent of the school-inspection and baby-health-station systems in the United States use duplicates of that system I perspired and agonized over because my newborn bureau was slowly suffocating under heaps and heaps of waste-paper. I did not want to pay out good money for pencils and carbon paper. But it was not the taxpayer I was thinking of—it was the babies who needed medicine and milk.

I was by no means the logical person for the job of constructing an organization for saving babies. It should have been in the hands of a person with all the theory and practice of governmental administration right at his fingers' ends. And I was just a harmless young woman from a small town who had been forced by circumstances into becoming a doctor for lack of any career that attracted her more. On the face of it I am still a doctor. In fact, when I took my degree as Doctor of Public Health in 1917, I became a doctor for the second time. But, largely by accident, I was forced into becoming an executive and having less and less to do with the practice of medicine. It is queer how, after the necessary jostling and shaking, you usually end up in the right spot. I was probably cut out to manage things, although it took me a long time to find it out. Whether I had started in a biscuit factory or a profession or a suburban kitchen, I would probably have ended up behind a desk somewhere making the telephone and a staff of assistants jump around in the interests of some widespread scheme or other. Perhaps that was why I so welcomed this venture into uncharted seas.

They *were* uncharted. No doubt it was just the right moment for some such experiment and someone else would have been starting it if we had not, but at that time the world was shockingly innocent of the kind of organization we found ourselves building. Only a few sporadic efforts of private organizations to solve certain aspects of the problem, such as the milk stations in Cleveland, Boston, Philadelphia, where modified milk for infant feeding was dispensed by private philanthropy to a handful of mothers, and school medical inspection of the most elementary type in a few cities. I have already given some idea of the inadequacy and slovenliness of school medical inspection as we found it. There was a badly administered child-labor law in New York State. That was all. Nothing coordinated, no governmental agency, federal, state, or municipal, which had been delegated any responsibility for children. A barbarous situation, when you look back on it from the vantage point of 1939. Eventually we took over the superintendence of the child's well-being from before birth till he turned the corner into adulthood.

When we started our campaign, we had a little knowledge developed out of our trial beginnings. The battle against infection in the worst schools was already well under way under a fine corps of nurses. The astonishing diminution in the baby death rate resulting from our attempt to educate slum mothers indicated a fertile field for further development. So we looked about for another point of attack, and decided that the midwives needed attention. Something had to be done about these women if far too many of our prospective charges were not going to be brought into the world maimed and blinded. And all that anybody knew about the midwife situation was that it was a crying scandal.

Although the midwife is as old as mankind, she was something of an anomaly in an American community, where the public had long been educated into the conviction that an M.D. and a hospital are the best combination for bringing children safely into the world. In New York thirty years ago, however, the huge recently landed immigrant population had kept the midwife tradition thoroughly alive. These Italian, Hungarian, Polish, Armenian, Greek, Slovak and other mothers had been accustomed to midwives in their native villages and wanted them here in the new country. They might not have been so badly off in experienced hands at home in the Balkans, but the New

[111]

York midwife was likely to be a very clumsy practitioner indeed who had got into the profession as an amateur and stayed in it to make a living. She was usually densely ignorant and therefore filthy, superstitious, hidebound, everything a good midwife should not be. Most of them eked out their scanty incomes from legitimate lyings-in by performing illegal operations under conditions that made you wonder how any of their patients survived. It was pretty grim business for these poor mothers who not only shrank from the idea of a man-doctor but couldn't afford him or a woman-doctor either.

Our first step was to install an efficient licensing system. The city had regulations requiring licenses, but enforcement was lax to the point of non-existence and proved nothing. No one knew how many midwives were practising or where or how. We went to the state legislature and secured new and stringent licensing laws for midwives in New York City, which were to be administered by the Department of Health. With the city in the picture, the midwives all had to come in and apply for licenses—a tremendous round-up—almost four thousand of them, I remember. They were all women of middle age or better, gabbling strange tongues, and dumb and frightened in the face of the fact that for the first time the law was checking up on them. They were too frightened to object to anything we wanted to do. Nevertheless, in order to gain their confidence and assure them we were not trying to run them out of business, we made the requirements easy. All you needed was a certificate from a doctor stating that you had been in attendance at twenty or more cases of childbirth under his supervision—something extremely easy to get. Everyone got a license, from the wrinkled old veteran who had had long experience in a Dalmatian hill town and probably knew as much about practical obstetrics as any doctor in New York, down to the shifty, filthy abortion-monger from Mott Street.

The medical profession, particularly the obstetricians, made a great deal of trouble for us at this point. Their idea was that the best thing would be to stamp out midwifery altogether instead of compromising with it. The doctors were never able to understand the sort of people we had to deal with. If deprived of midwives, these women would rather have amateur assistance from the janitor's wife or the woman across the hall than submit to this outlandish American custom of having in a male doctor for a confinement. Their daughters, the second generation of mothers, were a different matter, and learned to insist upon employing doctors as stubbornly as any American girl. We licensèd every midwife for the purpose of finding her address; after that it was a simple matter to deal with the ones who were unfit.

When they were accustomed to strict licensing, we began to require that future midwives earn the right to practice. Later, in 1911, a special midwives' school of obstetrics was started at Bellevue Hospital, and from then on we refused licenses to new applicants who were not graduates of either this school or a European school of equal standing. The Bellevue course, under city control, was for six months and free—but comprehensive and efficient, as it should have been. Its graduates knew more about delivering babies than three-quarters of the recently graduated internes entering on medical practice in this country that year. Then, when we started arresting and convicting some of the abortionists, most of the others moved to New Jersey or elsewhere, which weeded out the worst specimens and considerably reduced the number of midwives in practice. Before we began our work, midwives had been delivering about half the babies born in New York. Nowadays there are only about seven hundred of them in practice and they deliver less than a tenth of the annual births. A few years ago the Bellevue school was closed for lack of students.

I would not regard cutting down the number of trained midwives as necessarily a good thing under all circumstances. If I had a daughter who was going to have a baby, I would rather see her in the hands of one of those competent Scandinavian midwives who, in their own countries, work in squads under supervision of an obstetrician, than in the hands of the average general practitioner. A well-trained midwife deserves all possible respect as a practical specialist. It is by no means unlikely that the fact that the United States' maternal death rate is higher than that of any European country is predominantly due to American distrust of midwives. For, in the majority of instances, a first-class midwife has probably handled more maternity cases than any doctor except a veteran obstetrician. The obstetrician is, of course, the best possible person to bring a child into the world. But, since the economic factor rules him out in many cases, the midwife, who is not allowed to go beyond natural deliveries, often gives both mother and child a better chance than is possible with the over-use of anaesthesia and the mechanically assisted deliveries which some doctors use unskilfully in order to spare the patient pain.

I remember getting into a hot discussion with the New York Academy of Medicine on that point. I had published some figures which made it pretty clear that the maternal mortality rate from infection at the time of childbirth among mothers delivered in hospitals by doctors was far higher than among mothers delivered at home by mid-wives. Naturally that annoyed the Academy and I must admit that on the face of it, it made little sense. I had a very bad hour indeed sitting at an Academy meeting as the target of all kinds of pointed remarks—they did not exactly call me a liar, but they skirted around it much too close for comfort. Then, to prove their point, they started an investigation of their own. That was my innings. In preparing my figures I had been absurdly careful to make them as unfavorable as possible to my point of view. If a midwife had so much as walked into the room where a prospective mother was in bed, her death would be placed to the discredit of the midwife, even if it had occurred while the case was under the doctor's care. Since the Academy did not go into these details quite so carefully, their figures, when they were finally compiled, were even more favorable to the midwives than mine.

There is little doubt in my mind, that, until American students receive far more thorough training in obstetrics than they do now, the properly trained and properly super-vised midwife is a better practical obstetrician than a great many general practitioners have ever had a chance to be. It is not the doctor's fault. He is lucky if, upon entering practice, he has so much as been on hand during a few deliveries, let alone handled one himself. In other words, he may be equipped with only a rough, second-hand knowledge of the delicate technique involved. He does not particularly want obstetrical cases when he starts practice, except as a way of getting patients, because they are an immense amount of bother for relatively low fees. So, unless he decides to specialize in obstetrics, which is not the most glamorous or best-paying branch of medicine, he never gets that long course of baby after baby which eventually gives the midwife an uncanny skill in making deliveries normal everyday affairs.

But remember I am recommending only the well trained and well supervised midwife. It is still a disgrace that, in view of her possibilities as a practitioner for all but prosperous people, so little has been done about her in this country even now. There are whole regions of the United States, particularly in the South, where the midwife's status is still as irregular, hit-or-miss and consequently lethal as it was in New York when we started cleaning up the situation. Following our lead in these districts would be a long and dirty job for anybody who tried it, but thoroughly worth while if you admit that a baby has a right to be born whole.

The Crede technique—a drop of one percent silver nitrate in each eye immediately after birth to prevent gonorrheal infection—was required in all cases. When we started bringing the midwives under genuine regulation, there were hundreds and hundreds of children in New York blind asylums because no midwife had ever heard of Crede and probably would not have bothered with the drops if she had. We made every midwife telephone us at once if there was any sign of irritation in the eyes at all, and an inspector was sent immediately to make the diagnosis and to see that the baby had the appropriate care. A midwife lost her license if she did not use the drops in every case. But the silver nitrate solution they used did not work out satisfactorily. It was usually in a bottle in the midwife's kit, generally dirty and always evaporating up to a dangerous strength. So, among our other concerns, we had to invent a fool-proof, sanitary, convenient way of packing the solution. With the assistance of the Schieffelin laboratories we finally worked out a neat little package—

two beeswax capsules, each containing enough solution for one eye, packed in a little box with sterile needles for puncturing the capsules. One puncture, one squeeze into the eye and there you were. That little capsule is all over the world now. And, due to its religious use, cases of congenital blindness have practically disappeared in New York City.

That is a fair sample of the way we were always having to use our mother-wit and invent something which had not existed before because no one had taken into account the practical circumstances under which underprivileged children are born and brought up. When we started educating slum mothers in the necessity of ventilation, for instance, we ran into the unconquerable European prejudice on the subject of drafts and night air. An Italian or Roumanian mother knew, as certainly as she knew the sun was going to rise next morning, that to expose a room to outside air after dark was tantamount to suicide and she was pretty apprehensive about an open window between September and June in any case. Neither persuasion nor scolding succeeded; the open window was unattainable. So we had to think of some way of getting ventilation with closed windows. The answer proved to be a plain wooden board, its length the width of the window. Mrs. Galeazzi would consent to open her window if she could immediately fill the gap at the bottom with a comfortably impermeable board, and its appearance reconciled her to the fact that a certain amount of air was coming in between the sashes. A reasonable compromise, all things considered —and absolutely the best we could do until Mrs. Galeazzi's daughter grew up and became sufficiently Americanized to look on open windows with approval.

I even found myself turning couturière and designing

an entirely new system of baby clothes in order to reduce the slum mother's resistance to giving up her traditions of swaddling-bands and overdressing. An abdominal band, a shirt, a diaper, an underpetticoat and a dress was our old formula—involving three different occasions when the arms of a squirming baby had to be put through armholes. So I worked out the obvious but previously unthought-of system of making baby-clothes *all* open down the front and laying them out like a fireman's clothes before the baby appeared on the scene—dress wide open, petticoat on that with the armholes on top of the dress's sleeves, shirt on that, diaper down below all spread out, abdominal band on that—then you laid the baby on his back in the middle of it, put his arms through shirt, petticoat and dress in two motions, did up the band and diaper, buttoned everything, and there you were. The dress was made big in the shoulders and not as long as the three-foot baby-dress of those days, so that by the time the child was grown to the short dress stage, he had just about grown up to the same clothes. The whole idea worked so well in our affairs that the McCall Pattern Company heard of it and offered to try it on the world of prospective mothers in general. They sold sets of patterns for it and, at a royalty of a cent apiece, it made a very neat addition to a rising young woman's income. The Metropolitan Life Insurance Company ordered two hundred thousand of these patterns for distribution to their policy holders.

We had more rule-of-thumb practicality when the sickeningly high death rate in one of our largest foundling hospitals brought me up there to see what was wrong. I have never seen such a perplexing mystery as that place presented. The foundling babies were dying at the rate of about fifty percent—in other words, every other baby. Yet the death rate in the whole city, even before our work was well started, was only twelve percent in children below one year. And you could not possibly call it the hospital's fault. By that time I had acquired a flair for hospital inspection and there was apparently absolutely nothing wrong. Intelligent, well-trained nurses carrying out the last technique to the letter, absolute spotlessness and sanitation, approved feeding; nothing was wrong except that the babies were dying like flies, poor little wretches.

The hospital heads were understandably frantic. The only thing that occurred to me, as I turned this paradox over and over in my mind, was that the missing element, whatever it was, obviously had nothing to do with care from the hygienic point of view. Then something which had been vaguely in my mind for some time began to take definite form, something deriving from the curious fact that, although you could make big dents in the infant death rate in tenement districts, there did not seem to be much to do about the rate in wealthy districts. Sometimes it really looked as if a baby brought up in a dingy tenement room had a better chance to survive its first year, given reasonable care, than a baby born with a silver spoon in its mouth and taken care of by a trained nurse who knew all the latest hygienic answers. If you put those two together, you arrive at the same answer I did. I cannot say I exactly believed in it myself, but there was no other way of making sense of this foundling-hospital situation, so we tried it out.

We started taking these foundlings, every other one of whom was doomed to die before the year was out, and boarding them with tenement mothers—actually removing them from the admirable conditions of the hospital and exposing them to the hazards of slum conditions. Poor

mothers, who had already had experience in raising families under supervision of the Bureau of Child Hygiene,
were paid ten dollars a month to become foster mothers of
foundling babies until they were well started on the problem of staying alive. We chose our foster mothers carefully and gave them the necessary supervision and aid of
a trained staff of doctors and nurses, but even so we did not
expect the results we got. In four years we had only one
foundling in three dying where one in two had died before, and the decrease would probably have been much
sharper if we had had funds and facilities for boarding
them all out.

When we saw how successful this plan was, we really
went looking for difficulties and worked on the problem of
the hopeless ward in the foundling hospital, the place
where prematurely born and obviously moribund babies
were put and given the best of care. Thoroughly futile it
was : the death rate in that ward was actually one hundred
percent. Any scrawny, bluish, half-alive baby that went
there, to be wrapped in cotton wool and fed with a medicine dropper, was morally certain to fade out after a little
while, and through nobody's fault at all. There was no
possible harm in trying the foster-mother system on these
unfortunates, because they were all going to die anyway.
I went to the Russell Sage Foundation and induced them
to furnish an additional five dollars a month as pay for
foster mothers taking these difficult cases, and we began
moving these poor little potential ghosts out of this ward
where everything was light and sterile and spick and span,
into tenement rooms on Hester and Orchard streets. Off-
hand it sounds like murder. In actual practice, however,
the foster mothers worked miracles. We reduced the death

rate among these hopeless cases from practically one hundred percent to a little over fifty percent in one year.

It was just a guess on our part, an effort to alter an environment in order to give something better a chance to happen. But the more I reflected on the kind of alteration we had made, the closer I came to an idea which is, from the orthodox medical point of view, pretty heretical. There were the rich children, beautifully taken care of by white-starched professionals, dying with uncanny readiness as soon as something went wrong with them. There were the slum children who, given halfway proper feeding and care, could stand up under diseases that would have killed the rich children. There were the wretched little foundlings dying wholesale under fine hygienic conditions and flourishing, relatively anyway, when conditions were much worse—but, very significantly, when they began to get personal care from a maternally minded woman.

That was the chief difference and it meant something. The rich baby's nurse, who never picked him up and crooned to him, merely fed him the right thing at the right time and kept him properly aseptic, was in the same category as the foundling hospital's nurse who turned the foundling over at the right time and gave him the best of care with all the impersonal efficiency of a well-intentioned machine. That was why I became and still am a firm believer in mothering for babies: old-fashioned, sentimental mothering, the kind that psychologists decry. It should not be carried to excess and it should not be continued too long, but there is little doubt in my mind that many a baby has died for lack of it. He may still be unable to talk, walk or do anything but feed and cry and kick, but he nevertheless needs that sense of being at home in a new world which only fond personal attention from his mother or the psychological equivalent can give him. He needs it even more than he needs butterfat and fresh air and clean diapers. Modern medicine learned a good while ago to give him material things in greater quantity than ever before. But that he also needs the personal equation to give him a reason for living is the only answer I could ever find in that experience with the doomed foundlings.

Not that this is the only assignable reason for the relatively high mortality among the children of the well-to-do and the wealthy as opposed to those in the lower income brackets. The nearer the family income gets to $3,000 a year, the better chance a baby in that family has of living. The moment the family income crosses the $3,000 mark, the baby's chances of dying increase until the family income gets appreciably above that amount. This may well be because the lower income families are eligible for the kind of supervision and care that is given them by organizations like the Bureau of Child Hygiene. With sixty thousand babies a year under our care, we had a right to feel that this was true. The very wealthy mother can well afford to have proper prenatal care and careful supervision of her baby's life. I am tempted to say that she can afford to have the same care that is given freely to the poor. But the middle-class mother, neither rich nor poor, can seldom afford such care and is too proud to ask for it free. In this, as in nearly all other medical matters, the "white collar" class is unable to obtain the best of medical care or advice and the baby death rate tells the tale.

Another reason is that babies and children in the tenements acquire an immunity to disease from the very fact of their environment. This is not true of the better protected children of the rich. The whole question of this acquired immunity is a fascinating problem in medicine. Too much protection and care in avoiding the normal hazards of life can be a grave mistake. Three stories come to my mind which may help toward a better understanding of this complex immunity problem. The first is a personal experience. In my student days part of our experience came from work at Bellevue Hospital. Once, during the late spring, with other students, I was in the wards there making "rounds" with Dr. Alexander Lambert. It was just after Admiral Peary had returned from the North Pole and he had brought back with him a number of Eskimo men. Our pneumonia season was well over in New York and yet soon after their arrival, practically every one of these Eskimo men came down with a particularly virulent type of pneumonia and was being cared for in the hospital. So far as I can remember, nearly all of them died. They were not immune to this disease; it was unknown where they came from and so they were so susceptible that they succumbed at once.

The second and third stories are equally interesting. One was told me by Dr. William H. Welch of Johns Hopkins. He said that during the first months after the United States went into the World War, our soldiers in Europe consisted only of troops of the regular army, all men in splendid physical condition and with absolutely no trace of tuberculosis. These troops were quartered with troops from French Africa and soon afterward practically all of these Africans came down with tuberculosis in an acute and almost malignant form. They had never had tuberculosis at home; it was an unknown disease there. The mere contact with large numbers of men from a country where tuberculosis was endemic was sufficient; they were non-immune to this disease while the white men had acquired immunity by long contact with the infection. The last incident concerns the time of the World War also. When the troops from the small towns began coming to New York to be placed in camps nearby, these boys were promptly brought to the contagious disease hospitals of the New York City Department of Health suffering from the minor contagious diseases which we associate with childhood: measles, mumps, chicken pox and occasionally scarlet fever. Practically all of these country boys were our patients; they too had no immunity while our city boys either had had these diseases or had acquired immunity long since from living in a city where such diseases were always rampant.

So I do not think that anyone can take an undue share of credit for reducing the baby death rate when it takes place in the poorer districts. Still it had to be done and much to my surprise it was not at all difficult. The point that had to be stressed was its utter simplicity. Given a group of babies who were largely immune to the common infections and almost immune to conditions that would kill carefully brought-up children, we soon found that simple changes in diet, plenty of fresh air, simple clothing, adequate bathing and regular schedules worked wonders. Breast feeding alone is responsible for a large part of the reduction of the diarrhoeal diseases. Prevention of disease was not too difficult. It was extraordinarily easy to keep these babies well and the lowering death rate proved that this simple way was the right one to follow. We were helped enormously by the fact that we had to work out the right methods by trial and error. There was nothing that we could follow; we had to make our own way and evolve our own procedure, without precedents to help or to bother us. We had to go confidently into the practice of new techniques, had to improvise our own methods of midwife control and baby care. Our goal was to keep well babies well, so that they would not become sick and probably die, and we had to defy all orthodox methods when they did not bring us the desired results. Again it seems strange that the methods we evolved could ever have been new and untried.

We concentrated upon babies at first because reducing the baby death rate was, and still is, the most spectacular, the quickest and the easiest part of the whole field of child hygiene. When that was well established we moved on to the finally complete supervision of the whole cycle of child life.

CHAPTER VII

B ABY HEALTH STATIONS, AS WE CALLED THEM, were among the Bureau's earlier achievements and, as I look back on our work, were the place at which we first dug deep into the problems we had wished on ourselves.

At this point elder readers must cast their minds back thirty years or so and remember that in that short interval the whole milk supply of New York, and nearly all other big cities, has been revolutionized. The pasteurizing process was already known, but the great bulk of milk consumed by the poorer people was "grocery," or "loose" milk, unpasteurized, originating from all sorts and conditions of dairies, sold in dubious containers, and undoubtedly one of the most prolific sources of babies' and children's diseases. It came into New York City from six different states, all with different sanitary regulations and standards of enforcement, and was never less than twenty-four hours old when it entered the grocery store, to be dipped into for bulk sale. Under those circumstances telling a tenement mother to give her child so much milk a day was like telling her to give him a diluted germ-culture daily.

Then there was the other problem of how to get the tenement mother properly to modify cow's milk for the human baby. No modern mother needs to be told that the differences in protein and butter-fat content and other details between cow's and human milk are extremely important to the baby that drinks it. But that was new in our time too and had to be sold to the tenement mother, as only one of a number of things she must learn if she was not going to kill her baby even with the best intentions in the world.

In the baby health stations we were definitely building on the experience of others. France had developed private institutions called the *Goutte de Lait* and the *Consultation des Nourissons* which supplied milk for babies whose mothers had abandoned the idea of breast-feeding, making some attempt to teach modification, and in the United States, establishments generously subsidized by Nathan Straus and others were distributing modified and pasteurized milk free in some thirty large cities. (The Straus stations were gallant battlers in the cause of pasteurization and did a great deal to combat the public's unhappy prejudice against "cooked" milk.) But I think we were the first to use milk-distribution as a way of coming into contact with mothers in order to educate them in scientific child care—always modified by common sense as the cow's milk was modified for human babies' consumption. We early developed the idea that, if we sold whole milk just enough below standard prices to tempt mothers to come to us, we could teach these mothers a great deal about baby care in the process of milk-buying. "Women and children first" was our natural motto, and since young babies are helpless by definition, it was the women we campaigned for, first, last and always.

So we decided to set up in all of the poorer neighborhoods, Bureau establishments which would combine the education of mothers with the distribution of whole milk for young babies with instructions as to home modification. The eventual success of the scheme showed that it was thoroughly sound. But, when we put the idea up to the city fathers, they would have none of it. A fine notion, no doubt, but the tax rate was already at high-water mark and where would they get the money? Two years as head of the Bureau of Child Hygiene had already given me a lifetime of experience with municipal financiers, so I did not try to argue the point. If the city would not supply public funds, we would have to get private funds. With splendid public spirit Mrs. J. Borden Harriman formed a committee to raise enough money to start thirty baby health stations and keep them open for a few months. She raised about $165,000 from her wealthy friends and people in Wall Street, and this mechanism for supplying the babies of the poor with the necessity of life started to function on strictly capitalist money. Then, when the money ran out, I put it squarely up to the shrinking city fathers. Either the next budget included enough to keep these institutions going or they closed down, just when the wives and babies of thousands upon thousands of voters were beginning to value them and, which was probably even more pertinent, just when the newspapers were waxing most enthusiastic about the stations' good work. Due in great measure to the influence of George McAneny, who was President of the Board of Aldermen under the reform administration of Mayor Mitchel, the city fathers managed to see the point. When all the parliamentary rubbish was cleared away we had an appropriation large enough for all our old stations and ten additional new ones. We all smiled at one another and started in to lease new premises and paint them blue, yellow and white—nice clean colors which also happened to be the colors of the city flag. They were well equipped and furnished.

Like everyone else in the medical profession of the day,

I had been trained in the then unimpeachable Rotch school of milk-modification, which was based on consideration of the baby's age, health, complexion, nationality, color of eyes and numerological and astrological data—or at least so it seemed when you started working with it. Pediatricians insisted that no tenement mother, lacking accurate instruments and technical training, could do anything at all with milk-modification, and with that method they were quite right, so private milk stations of the Straus type had previously modified the milk for each mother, establishing a special laboratory for that purpose. But with *our* overcrowded facilities that method would have been like trying to serve a nine-course banquet for five hundred people out of a kitchenette. So I risked my professional reputation and all my hopes of getting cooperation from the medical profession, who were already quite sufficiently upset about the possible effects of our free service upon private practice, by starting a scheme for modifying milk which threw out all the higher mathematics and complications of the Rotch method and put the addition of water, lime-water and milk-sugar on the simple basis of what the baby weighed. I was not so presumptuous as to do it alone. Three eminent pediatricians sat in on the preparation of these formulae. But they were so apprehensive about it that they solemnly pledged me to keep their names out of it when the storm broke. It broke. Once again high and mighty medical associations called me a murderer and once again I was able to demonstrate with figures that the babies I was murdering were much livelier little ghosts than the city had ever known before. Today that system of milk-modification is standard practice everywhere for well babies.

But that is by the way. The emphasis was on the fact

that Mrs. Slivowitz was coming to the baby health station
—*with her baby*—having it given a careful examination
and receiving a cheerily disguised lesson in how to care
for it, and then taking her quart of milk home to modify
it herself. I remember one tenement mother who con-
fessed to a visiting nurse that her baby, a poor little wretch
with all kinds of skin ailments, had never been bathed
since she had left the hospital with him. When she was
asked why: "I can't bathe him," she said, "I haven't got
any marble slab at home." And then it came out that the
only time the poor soul had ever seen her child bathed
had been in the hospital on a marble slab, which, she had
concluded, was as essential a part of the procedure as soap
and water. Everything you taught had to be simple and
standardized enough to fit that kind of mentality.

That was a fairly successful job of hewing to the line,
and the chips had not wrought any permanent damage, no
matter how angry they made people for the moment. All
during the development of our organization the Department of Health had also been working on the problem of
the milk supply. When the smoke had all cleared away,
New York City had established the familiar *A*, *B* and *C*
standards of milk grading which now make it practically
certain that the consumer gets pure milk for his money.
A milk is either certified raw milk, free from all suspicion
of contamination, or the richest kind of pasteurized milk.
B is a perfectly respectable pasteurized milk, which makes
up the bulk of present-day consumption, and it must be
bottled before delivery to store or customer. *C* is not necessarily pasteurized or bottled and so can be used only for
industrial purposes; it is against the law to sell it for drinking purposes. As I mentioned before, the public was
vaguely hostile to the idea of pasteurized milk, and I must

confess that, before the dairies perfected the process, pasteurizing the milk did make it taste as though it had been boiled. It hardly needs to be mentioned that the big milk companies were against pasteurization because the process was expensive and called for an installment of new equipment and eternal care. But the public was gradually sold on, and the companies gradually forced into, the idea. In no time the public was drawing huge dividends of health. (I do not mean that all this was due to the work of the Bureau of Child Hygiene. We were only one of hundreds of organizations in the campaign for safe milk.) Our supply was early arranged with the Sheffield Company, from a specially selected creamery out beyond Port Jervis. This milk was of Grade *A* quality, pasteurized and bottled at the dairy, brought into the city on ice in special cars, and delivered each morning only a few hours after the milking. They established a price which enabled us to sell Grade *A* to our mothers at the same price they would have paid for Grade *B* at the store.

At first we concentrated our efforts on cajoling mothers into coming to buy bargain milk from us and learning how to modify it for the baby's uses. They were not very keen on the idea; we could not have induced them to buy the milk from us without that three-cent difference in price. But, as soon as a few mothers began to see the difference in their babies, they were only too glad to come to our stations. They say it takes word-of-mouth advertising to make a hit of a play or a movie—that is just as true of any public welfare project. Mrs. Slivowitz told the woman across the air-shaft who passed it on to the janitor's wife and so it went up and down the block like a contagious disease. Presently our hard-working staff of nurses had to stop their canvassing of suspicious tenement mothers because the stations were swamped. It was a beautiful case of snowballing: during my latter years in office we were caring for 60,000 babies a year. And they flourished like so many green bay trees.

By the time we began developing the Little Mothers' League idea, we knew enough to start the work in terms of prevention without waste motion. The fundamental idea of this development came to me in 1910 when I read a book by John Spargo called "The Bitter Cry of the Children," all about the "little mother" and what a menace she was to society as a fertile source of infant mortality. The "little mother" is the girl child of the poor, forced by poverty to take over the care of the next-youngest child because her mother is struggling to hold down the job that feeds the whole family. I understand that the little-mother system works out very well in the remoter islands of the Samoan group—is, in fact, the basis of the whole Samoan tradition of child care. But Orchard Street in New York City is not Samoa and the hygienic emergencies of bringing up a child in an east side gutter are not the same as those in a culture composed of clean sea-water and palm-groves.

No one had to tell me about the little mother of the New York slum. I had seen her much too often myself—a scrawny child of eight or nine, dirty and dishevelled, lugging a dirtier and more dishevelled baby which alternated between peevish wailing and sucking at something anonymous, crying all the louder when the little mother slapped it in understandable childish impatience with the nagging noise. But I could not dodge the issue by merely agreeing with Mr. Spargo's point that there should be no such thing as a little mother, innocently and ignorantly killing her thousands of children a year. That was not our slant on things. We could not afford the luxury of saying things should or should not be. We had to work realistically with the raw materials and situations at hand. Since thousands of poor families were in an economic situation which made the little mother necessary, we had to turn her into something that suited our purpose.

Public school was the obvious point of contact. These girl-children, prematurely saddled with maternal responsibilities, were mostly of school age and the truant-officer made certain that they were in the schoolroom. If the schools would install classes in practical child-hygiene— for whether little mothers or not, most of these girls would eventually become mothers in their own right—our problem would be solved. But the educational authorities did not even bother to laugh at me when I made the suggestion. Reading, writing, arithmetic, manual training, gymnastics—but not child care, that process through which everybody goes and which all women should know as they know how to dress themselves. It was many years later that, in view of the success of our Little Mothers' Leagues in New York, Chicago installed public school courses in child care which made Little Mothers' Leagues happily pointless.

When I got my thick-headed refusal from the New York educational authorities, I went directly to Miss Margaret Knox, the principal of Public School 15, with far more enterprise and imagination than her superiors, and had no difficulty at all in getting her to sponsor the first Little Mothers' League in her school. Whether the Board of Education had endorsed the idea or not, school after school fell into line and in no time, just to simplify my task of pioneering in child welfare at the same time that I was running a flourishing private medical practice, I had

[133]

a flock of Little Mothers' Leagues to care for, though my staff shouldered most of the burden.

Children are natural "joiners." If there is nothing else to join, they will form mystic secret societies of their own or street-corner gangs. Added to that is the girl-child's irrepressible impulse to play mother—with a doll—if she is fortunate, with a live baby if economic handicaps require it. It was a revelation of the fundamental strength of the mothering instinct that having to look after their younger brothers and sisters had not spoiled these little mothers' eagerness to learn child care as a fascinating game. A Little Mother, with her unwearying desire to make the world more habitable for babies attested by her gold-washed badge of honor awarded as recognition of constant attendance at meetings, had in no time at all become as cheering an object as it has ever been my lot to witness.

Once the Leagues were started, in simple groups taking practical instruction from nurses in baby feeding, baby exercising, baby dressing and the other parts of baby care, they branched out in directions no one had thought of. These youngsters were among our most efficient missionaries, canvassing tenements for us, cajoling mothers of their acquaintance into giving the baby health stations a trial, checking up on mothers who had backslid in attendance at the stations, telling every mother they met all about what they were learning. They organized fresh-air outings for their own mothers and babies, proudly taking all responsibility for both during a whole day in the country or a trip down the harbor on the St. John's Guild boat. For the benefit of groups of mothers, they wrote and acted wonderful plays, half mediaeval mystery-play and half vaudeville skit. The favorite plot introduced a crying baby, screaming its head off, and a harassed mother who has no notion whatever of what to do about it. Enter several neighbors, some sympathetically distressed about the mother's troubles, some furious because the baby is keeping them awake, all making a terrific hubbub with unintelligent suggestions. Just when you are wondering why somebody does not turn in a police riot-call, enter a Little Mother who sizes up the situation at a glance and settles everything by inspecting the baby and removing an open safety pin which has caused all the disturbance. Then, of course, she delivers a practical demonstration of just what to do with babies under any and all conceivable circumstances, and the play closes, with the Little Mothers in the cast bursting with pride in their own superior knowledge and the mothers in the audience vividly impressed with new ideas about fresh air and soap and water.

"Hear Not the Advice of a Neighbor; or How Babies Die" was the tragic title of one of these propaganda playlets of our Little Mothers. And here is the complete text of a short playlet for the curious in such matters—not a triumph of dramaturgy but certainly very much to the point:

MOTHER: Baby wants something to eat.
CHILD: What?
MOTHER: I guess a piece of pineapple.
CHILD: Mother, what! Pineapple for a baby?
MOTHER: What's the matter?
CHILD: You do not mean pineapple for a baby, do you?
MOTHER: Yes, I think baby will like a piece very much.
CHILD: No matter if the baby will like it or not it is not healthy for babies.
MOTHER: Who told you that?

CHILD: I belong to the Little Mothers' League. They teach us how babies ought to be kept.

MOTHER: You did not tell me that. I would have stopped giving it to the baby a long time ago.

CHILD: I'll tell you what they taught me: how to clean bottles, how to make barley water, and how the babies ought to be taken care of during the summer. You see, mamma, that the doctor in our school is very kind to take a part of the Saturday to teach that to us.

MOTHER: Baby seems to be getting fatter and better every day since I stopped giving it fruit and the things you told me were not good for the baby.

CHILD: You see that our club is of good use.

MOTHER: Thanks ought to be given to the doctor of your school.

And on another occasion when we asked the Little Mothers each to draw up her list of twelve "don'ts" for mothers of young children we found some startling prohibitions among the number: "Don't give the baby herring"; "Don't give the baby beer to drink"; "Don't leave the baby run in the mud-gutter"; "Don't let the baby eat dirty things from the floor that she threw down at first; also pickle"; "Don't scream on the baby"; "Don't try to awaken its intelligence and make it laugh"; "Don't leave the baby alone in the carriage and play with your friends" (aimed straight at Little Mothers as well as fashionable nursemaids); "Don't give the baby sour cucumbers"; and, as a lurid touch which probably recalls some harrowing experience of the family next door: "Don't leave the baby sit on the stove"; and, for finale, "Don't mind your house —mind your children." Weird as they are, there is a healthy realism and a solid sense of tenement conditions about these terse bits of advice which still assures me that we trained our Little Mothers pretty well and that they had a lot of common sense of their own to start with.

Naturally we encountered opposition to our Little Mothers' Leagues. There is always opposition to anything worth doing. The ignorant and the malicious—it often amounts to the same thing—protested that we were making premature slaves of these children so that their mothers could slide out of their responsibilities and go off to the movies or get drunk. But gradually we induced most people to see that, since the little mother was an inevitable makeshift, she would be far less dangerous to her charges if she were intelligently trained. When letters began to pour in on us from everywhere, not only from this country, Europe and South America, but from India, China, Turkey and Japan, asking us how to start similar movements, we knew that our justification was complete. You seldom cause international sensations with schemes that are fundamentally unsound.

There was a great deal of discouragement involved in this process of getting the politicians, the public, the whole body of mothers and the medical profession to take up a new idea and carry it out with intelligence and efficiency. I think that, of the whole list, the medical profession made the least intelligent difficulties. As an M.D. in good standing, a veteran of years of private practice and a member of several first class medical societies, I can say that without any suspicion of speaking out of turn. I have a tremendous respect for my profession as a whole and for thousands of its individual members with whom I have worked and to whom I have gone with my own physical ailments. But any large body of people grouped by common interests will never behave with a tenth the intelligence that its individual members will show in their daily lives. That is true of nations, street-corner gangs, prayer-meetings—and large groups of doctors.

I have already described two or three occasions when my colleagues insisted on getting in our way for what seemed to us the worst of all possible bad reasons. But I never saw the short-sighted psychology of a certain type of doctor, when confronted with public health work, better brought out than by a representative of a New England medical society testifying before a Congressional committee which was considering the appropriation of funds for the newly founded Federal Children's Bureau. I was down there testifying too—on the other side. This New England doctor actually got up and told the committee: "We oppose this bill because, if you are going to save the lives of all these women and children at public expense, what inducement will there be for young men to study medicine?" Senator Sheppard, the chairman, stiffened and leaned forward: "Perhaps I didn't understand you correctly," he said; "You surely don't mean that you want women and children to die unnecessarily or live in constant danger of sickness so there will be something for young doctors to do?" "Why not?" said the New England doctor, who did at least have the courage to admit the issue; "That's the will of God, isn't it?"

Those Congressional hearings were usually productive of something worth remembering. I was always going down to testify at hearings on Children's Bureau appropriations because Miss Julia Lathrop, the Bureau's brilliant first chief, thought I was a good ally. I was called Doctor instead of Miss and so could escape from the eternal remark always coming up among Congressmen about giving money to an old-maid to spend. I remember one occasion when the pending bill about funds for child welfare, for some reason which I could only conclude was a bad pun that somebody had taken seriously, had been referred to the House Committee on Labor. It was a hundred and ten in the shade, a fine, bracing summer morning in Washington and, to spare the committee, I suggested that they should ask me questions instead of letting me make a speech that would probably smother us all with boredom. As it was we nearly all went to sleep anyway—that is the only way I can account for the fact that when, in answer to a question, I said that there were six maternity deaths for every thousand labors, a Congressman spoke up angrily. "Now come, come, doctor," he said, "we're not going to bring labor into this. There's too much talk about the laboring-man anyway."

Nevertheless it was not impossible to get a certain stimulation out of stupid opposition, whether political or professional. Charts and statistics gave the Bureau staff encouragement inside the office as things started working. But the city at large did not comprehend what we were after for quite a while and that tended to make us feel pretty blue at times. I remember how I felt when, after we had our baby health stations established and doing well in the Brownsville section of Brooklyn, a petition was forwarded to my desk from the Mayor's office, signed by thirty-odd Brooklyn doctors, protesting bitterly against the Bureau of Child Hygiene because it was ruining medical practice by its results in keeping babies well, and demanding that it be abolished in the interests of the medical profession. I was feeling pretty low that day—something urgent had gone wrong and I had been wondering if all this trouble we were going to was just so much waste motion. That petition cheered me up like a cocktail. I reached for a pen and endorsed it in great big letters:

"This is the first genuine compliment I have received since the Bureau was established. I am profoundly grateful for having had an opportunity to see it,"—and sent it back to the Mayor's office in a hurry.

I never heard of it again. But it had had its tonic effect. The only thing that would have done better would have been a similar protest from an undertakers' association.

The work itself occasionally suffered from the blundering of doctors to whom it had never occurred that, if you went about things with insufficient preparation, you were likely to provoke riots among parents and children who would have been amiable enough if intelligently handled. In our tonsil-and-adenoid riot, for instance, I found myself in accord with the rioters. That was the culmination of several years of trying to make operable tonsil-and-adenoid cases in the public schools fit into our limited facilities for taking care of them. Hospital clinics were being swamped with cases referred by school medical inspectors, and post-operative treatment was out of the question; time and again I was called up in the middle of the night to reassure a frightened nurse about another case of post-operative septic sore throat or haemorrhage. It was not my line—I was a pediatrician, not a nose-and-throat specialist—but anyone working with a Bureau of Child Hygiene has to know a good deal about everything that can go wrong with human beings, except possibly senile dementia.

Since the clinics were so overworked, a brilliant staff member in a big hospital suggested that the doctors would do far better to go around and perform tonsil-and-adenoid operations *en masse* in the schools themselves instead of cluttering up the clinics. The Bureau knew nothing about this decision. I first heard of it when I got a 'phone call that there was serious trouble at one of the public schools on the lower east side and went down to investigate. The school yard was clogged with a mob of six or seven hundred Jewish and Italian mothers wailing and screaming in a fine frenzy and apparently just on the point of storming the doors and wrecking the place. Every few minutes their hysteria would be whipped higher by the sight of a child ejected from the premises bleeding from mouth and nose and screaming with sheer panic. In view of what I saw when I had fought my way inside, I would not have blamed the mothers if they had burned the place down. For the doctors had coolly descended on the school, taken possession, lined the children up, marched them past, taken one look down each child's throat, and then two strong arms seized and held the child while the doctor used his instruments to reach down into the throat and rip out whatever came nearest to hand, leaving the boy or girl frightened out of a year's growth and bleeding savagely. No attempt at psychological preparation, no explanation to the child or warning to the parents. In ten seconds I was in the middle of it, shouting that it must stop at once. When that point was carried, and it required a good deal of pointed language to carry it, I turned to pacifying the mob of mothers and getting them to go home. It was an outrage—as cruel and as stupid as an initiation ceremony in an African tribe. You would have thought these children were so many fox-terriers having their ears and tails clipped, and that does not mean I approve of clipping them either.

It was stopped all right—stopped so short that there were no more of these operations done in school buildings. But with the overcrowded conditions in the clinics, the next move was up to me. I brought the matter up at the next meeting of the Section on Laryngology of the Academy of Medicine. What I wanted was assurance that, instead of this wholesale slaughter of innocents which, I shrewdly suspected, included many cases which did not need operations at all, the hospitals would take all justifiable school cases, give them a skilled operator, use approved anaesthetics and supply twenty-four hours of postoperative care before sending the child home. I said that, if they would not cooperate to that reasonable extent, I would open our own hospitals. The assembled laryngologists took that for mere bluster and said "No."

So I bided my time, caught the city fathers in a melting mood and obtained an appropriation for six small hospitals, city-run, specializing in nose-and-throat operations, staffed by men from our own medical force who were sent to get special training in this sort of work. They were beautiful little hospitals, with the latest equipment and surpassing technical standards. Then we started sending to them all school cases that were really operable, bringing in the children the evening before, operating under nitrous oxide gas and oxygen in the morning, keeping them all day surrounded by toys and ice cream and sending them home fit and cheerful that night. In six years we removed thousands upon thousands of adenoids and tonsils without a single fatality or a single instance of septic sore throat or post-operative bleeding—that last due in no small measure to our routine use of the new "thromboplastin" which had just been perfected by Dr. Alfred Hess. Our one difficulty was of a gratifying kind: the children had such a good time that it was sometimes a task to get them to go home. These hospitals were maintained for about five years. Then the general hospitals of the city agreed to follow the same procedure and we gladly turned the work back to them.

The small but all-important details of human nature's

peculiarities never left us alone. They were usually our worst enemies till we began to understand and turned them into allies. Even in something so obviously insignificant as the name of an organization. Back in 1909, when our work at the Bureau was just getting solidly under way, a group of child hygiene people, myself included, decided to form an association for the exchange and promotion of child welfare ideas. We called ourselves, at some length, "The American Association for the Study and Prevention of Infant Mortality." It was a small organization, but vigorous, and usually lacking funds in its early days. Presently we had a meeting in Boston's Faneuil Hall and the Mayor of Boston, an astute politician by definition, introduced me when I made my speech. He had a terrific struggle with that interminable name and gave it up in despair. Afterward, he said to me:

"I'm always glad to welcome people to Boston, doctor. But if you don't change the name of your society, I am never going to welcome you here again. And by the way," he went on, "do you have trouble raising money?" I said that we usually did. "It's that name," he said. "Nobody is going to write anything as long as that on a check. By the time they get halfway through, they will change their minds." There is a lesson in that for a good many long-named societies.

That was one of the reasons why we changed the name to "The American Child Hygiene Association." The "Child" came in naturally for we were extending its interests, and our own, to cover the field of childhood. One of the things I learned early was that you cannot separate the child into categories. The baby's health is dependent upon the pre-natal period; healthy babies become healthy pre-school children; health in school children is largely dependent upon the years that have gone before, and adult health is mainly dependent upon health during the whole period of childhood. The child had to be taken as a whole; if we divided our efforts into work for different age-groups it was just for efficiency: every period of the baby's or child's life was bound up with every other period.

The American Child Hygiene Association was a vigorous and inspiring society. I later became its president, and during my entire career there was no other organization that gave me so much of the association of people of like minds and interest and inspiration. In 1923, when Herbert Hoover became its president, it amalgamated with The Child Health Organization of America, which had been founded a few years before by Dr. L. Emmett Holt, the eminent author of that mothers' Bible, *The Care and Feeding of Children*. The combined organization, as "The American Child Health Association," was dissolved only in 1935, merging in one direction with The National Education Association and in the other with The American Public Health Association. Through its many years of work and its many changes in name, it was a tower of strength to all who were interested in child health. That fact, that there seems no longer to be a need for organizations of that specialized type, is a tribute to the firm establishment of child hygiene work today.

I know how dreary it is to look down the list of organizations for this and that and how easy it is to wonder what they are all about and why they exist. There are far too many, without doubt; and of committees on various subjects there is no end. I resigned from twenty-six committees when I retired, and I might have belonged to many more with little effort. In some curious way, these committees seemed always to be made up of much the same people:

Lillian Wald, Annie Goodrich and I seemed to be peripatetic members of most of them. I remember one night when one of these committees was meeting in the United Charities Building, our door was suddenly flung open and a reporter from *The Sun* looked in. "What are you calling yourselves tonight?" was his greeting. But in my field, at least, organizations were the breath of life. In order to get cooperation from all types of people, I had advisory committees on every conceivable phase of my work. Someone has said that a committee is an organization that takes three months to do what any able-bodied man can accomplish in half an hour. They took a great deal of time out of life, were usually tiresome, only occasionally helpful, but they gave the members a sense of importance that made them cooperative and so they seemed to be worth while.

But I founded one organization of which I have always been proud. It still exists and is a most valuable part of our city's affairs. This started as "The Association of Baby Health Stations." When we started our baby health stations, we found three other private organizations already in the field. One was the Nathan Straus Milk Stations, another the Diet Kitchen, under the presidency of Mrs. Henry Villard, and the third a group of baby milk-dispensaries financed and managed by Mrs. Adrienne Joline. In order that we might not duplicate the work of one another, I asked them to meet with me and form this little organization. They were all most cooperative and for a year or more the society functioned in this small way. The New York Milk Committee paid the salary of a secretary and the Department of Health furnished an office, stenographic aid and postage. In a short time it was evident that the same sort of cooperative concern was needed for older children. In this latter field, there was serious overlapping of work and much confusion. So our little group became "The Children's Welfare Federation" and so remains to this day.

The Children's Welfare Federation is a clearing house for the city for all organizations which touch the welfare of the child. It was, so far as I have been able to discover, the first organization which drew together the functions of all sorts of allied agencies. Under the direction of Miss Mary Arnold, who was its most efficient secretary, it has served a great need and can be turned to at any time to find the right organization for any type of child care from pre-natal work to psychiatry. Now, no child need longer have her ear syringed six times each day by the nurses from three organizations; now no baby need die while its mother waits until someone can find a hospital to receive it; now no baby need go without breast milk and no child need lack a vacation. Today over two hundred and fifty organizations belong to the Children's Welfare Federation and this type of organization exists in practically all of the large communities in the United States.

That was the gradually encouraging thing about the whole development of the Bureau of Child Hygiene. There was a lot of stupidity, a great deal of waste motion, much ignorance to be combated, but always the enthusiasm and devotion of the doctors and nurses of the Bureau. The idea was good; we tried to work it out with common sense, and through the mass of detail and discouragement it was spreading. People didn't really like to see children die.

Chapter VIII

I LIKE TO REMEMBER THE AMUSING EPISODES OF my life; possibly because they stood out in contrast to the alternating monotony and difficulties of most days. At the time, my work seemed super-exciting, but as I look back over the years they seem to have merged into each other and to have flowed onward like days on shipboard, without beginning and without end and much alike in their seemingly endless, unbroken progression. The good was mixed with the bad; the funny with the serious. But that, of course, is common to all lives.

Some of the most joyous interludes were caused by the letters that used to come to the school nurses from mothers of children who had been sent home with some physical defect or other. One proved very valuable for publicity purposes. It was reproduced in several magazines and innumerable newspapers and attributed to many and varied sources. But we had the original note. The boy was sent home because he was so obviously in need of a bath. The letter from the mother came promptly: "Dear Teacher," it read, "Ikey aint no rose. Don't smell him—learn him." There was less imagination but a considerable sense of emphatic rhetoric about this one: "Dear Nurse: As for his nose, it don't need it. As for his tonsils, he was born with them. As for his teeth, he'll get new ones. Please mind your own business."

To the time when we were giving the Schick test to

children to determine the presence of immunity to diphtheria, belongs this gem (it may be remembered that the year 1922 was just about the high water mark of Rudolph Valentino's popularity in "The Sheik") : "Dear Teacher: I've read the book and I've seen the movie and I don't want my boy to have none of it." And I remember vividly an irate mother who came to my office and demanded to see me. She brandished one of the printed forms used by the nurses: "What does this mean?" she demanded. "My boy is as bright as any." I took the form; it was evident the nurse was a time-saver, for instead of "poor nutrition" she had written "poor nut."

These experiences serve as avenues for me to look down as I think back over this incredibly complicated task of trying to assure health to one million, two hundred thousand school children. I may laugh when I think of these stories but they also carry me back to the tangled problem of school medical inspection. We met and mastered the almost overwhelming occurrence of contagious eye and skin diseases; we did our share in reducing the incidence of the ordinary contagious diseases common in child life, but we never made any impression upon the problem of physical defects so common during childhood and, so far as I know, that problem has never been even faintly solved by anyone. Since its inception, school medical inspection has cost untold millions of dollars and received the earnest attention of the greatest experts in the child health field. It is still a dismal failure and this money might have been spent with better results in almost any other field of public health.

Perhaps that problem has always haunted me because it was the inefficient horrors of school medical inspection which constituted my initiation into public health work. I assisted at its birth and then followed the poor little thing throughout its entire anaemic history, and my opinion of its validity is much the same today as it was when I first encountered its forlorn beginnings. Because of the great expense of this work, its major importance in public health and its entire failure, I shall speak again about it at greater length. Here I can only refer to the belief that we must have more and more doctors and nurses, that we must cover a larger and larger field and that we must convince more and more parents of the vital necessity of having their children's physical defects remedied. Other cities have followed this line of thought and, when money was forthcoming, increased their forces, still with no appreciable results. Several cities, failing to get the necessary appropriations, speeded up their work, announced a physical examination of every child every year and made a farce of the whole proceeding. The statistics were sickeningly commonplace in the way in which they repeated themselves.

In New York City, it was economically impossible to induce the city fathers to appropriate enough money to provide for an annual physical examination. The fantastic expense involved made us try to compromise on an examination when the child entered school, another about the fourth grade and the final one when the child was ready to leave school. The trouble was that we were not dealing in babies this time. The mere name, "baby," holds a rhetorical and emotional appeal that will touch the heart of even the most hardened holder of the city's purse strings. But there was no comparable way to dramatize the older children's failing vision, decayed teeth and diseased lungs. Parents, as a class, were far from cooperative. We would send the child home with a card telling of the physical defect found and asking the mother to take her child to her doctor, get his advice and then report back to the nurse. The returns were so disappointing that we appealed to the medical profession in general. We devised a new system by which the original examination could be made by the family physician and a report sent to us. This meant a vast saving in expenditure of money and we hoped for a big response. In the earliest years about sixteen percent of the examinations were done by the family doctor. And then the mothers began to realize that they did not have to spend their own money for this purpose. Gradually, the whole burden was shifted back to our overworked staff. There was no way to defeat the natural human instinct to refuse to pay for anything you can get free.

And overworked our doctors and nurses certainly were. There seemed so much to be done and so little time to do it. The pressure from the Board of Education and even from the Department of Health itself was a driving force. I had my strong suspicion that our examinations were very superficial and of little account. We did not undress the children and only too often there were innumerable layers of clothing to hide their bodies and make listening difficult. A large and powerful organization interested in child welfare began publicly reproaching us for inefficiency, on the ground that we could not be doing efficient physical examinations without undressing the children. To quiet them, I apprehensively instructed a few of the staff, all women, to undress the girls and always to have the nurse or mother present when this was done. And then another storm broke. At least two of the New York newspapers chose to make front page news, with glaring headlines, of stories of schoolgirls being insulted and stripped by brutal Health Department doctors, all broadcast with pictures of the insulted girls and much journalistic indignation. An investigation immediately exploded these ridiculous charges but we could not go on with this method. We had to do the best we might with the children fully dressed. I then asked committees of specialists to go about the schools and check up on our examinations. When the figures of their results were given to me, I was immensely cheered to find that with the same children, the results of our staff and of these efficient doctors varied by hardly a fraction of one percent. Even the heart specialists were startlingly close in their findings to the results of our staff examinations though heart lesions are notoriously difficult to diagnose even without clothing to mask the sounds.

We might be fairly sure that our diagnoses were accurate but getting these children treated was a totally different matter. The basic theory of public health work precludes any treatment of a disease unless it is a contagious disease which may become a public menace. When one considers that the greater part of our children came from families who had no excess money and that their physical defects were not too prominent, it was exceedingly difficult to induce these parents to pay some doctor to treat an ailment that seemingly did not cripple the child. The nurses would make from two to twelve visits to each of these homes; they would offer to take the children to a free clinic. But either fear or plain neglect offered a sufficient rebuff. With every effort we could make, we could rarely get more than thirty-five percent of the children treated and this thirty-five percent represented a very much smaller fraction of the total number of children in the schools who needed attention. It was disheartening work and I am sure our experience was duplicated in every medical inspection system in the country. Nor have matters improved since the early days; the proportion of children who are cared for in any adequate manner still remains disturbingly low.

Later we turned more and more to public health education to prepare the way. It was far easier to induce a mother to adjust the artificial light so that her child's eyes might not be strained when reading, to teach families how to give their children the proper food and rest that might prevent undernourishment and to break their prejudice against night air in bedrooms, than to start with an ignorant mind to combat and demand immediate medical treatment. Our diplomatic method of approach when the Schick test was first introduced may stand as an example of the way we sought to induce mothers to try some measure of child care. The chief point of leverage is always the fact that, although the average mother will go a long way with you, she does so only when she is convinced in her own mind that whatever is proposed will be good for her child. We were working among an almost wholly foreign population; today, with the restricted immigration and the building up of a more American citizenry, it may not be so difficult as it used to be. But I doubt if ignorance, fear and neglect can be considered as belonging to any racial group. We are all a little apprehensive of the unknown. And, other things being equal, the younger the child the more the mother will try to protect it against intrusive strangers with curious ideas.

When Dr. William H. Park, then director of the Bureau of Laboratories of the Department of Health, wished to start a drive to make the Schick test as nearly universal as possible, he asked my staff to cooperate in carrying on the actual work. We started by giving the test to the school children after having obtained the parents' permission in

each instance. When a child was found to be non-immune
to diphtheria we immunized him with routine injections of
toxin-antitoxin. Today toxin is used for this purpose. We
knew we were wrong from the scientific and statistical
points of view. It may be more spectacular to immunize
the children of school age but they are not the ones who
need it most nor is their age the one when this immuniza-
tion will do the most good. We should have concentrated
on babies, for that is the susceptible period for diphtheria.
The time of highest non-immunity lies in the period between six months and two years of age after the baby has
lost his mother's adult immunity and before he has had a
chance to acquire it for himself. But preventive public
health work, as well as the group we should have reached,
was then in its infancy and we had to prepare the way in
a devious fashion. We parted company with sense and
science here. We knew we should have a fearful battle inducing mothers to let us test their babies, whereas permission to test older children was more easily gained. When
a mother had once known her older child to come through
such a test unharmed and when, after the subsequent injections of toxin-antitoxin she was convinced that her child
was protected against diphtheria, it was not too difficult for
her to let her baby have the Schick test too.

The Bureau of Child Hygiene did its share in reducing
the toll of the general contagious diseases. We had only a
vague relationship with the home quarantine of these
cases; our function was to protect the child while he was
in school. When we began our work, measles, scarlet fever,
chicken pox, mumps and whooping cough were all famil-
iarly known as "school diseases." At least we have changed
that designation. They may still be called "diseases of the
school age" but the school itself has lost the stigma of

being responsible for their occurrence and spread. As a matter of fact, with any adequate system of health control in the schools, they may well be the safest places where a child can go during any epidemic. The teachers cooperated with us nobly in this campaign. In groups, they were instructed, not in diagnosis of the various diseases, but in the detection of "something wrong" physically. Each morning, each teacher looked over the children in her class. If any showed any symptom of flushed face, obvious cough, listlessness or a rash, that child was sent at once to the doctor's office in the school and told to wait there until he came and could decide whether the child might go back to the classroom or must be sent home. A report to the Department office in each suspicious case brought another inspector who might at leisure make the final diagnosis and enforce quarantine if a contagious disease was found. Simple enough, but surprisingly effective in its results. It is interesting to know how the character of some of these diseases has changed. Years ago, scarlet fever was considered a deadly disease; today it is almost innocuous. On the other hand measles, which was formerly thought of as a necessary part of child life and of little consequence, is now a serious disease. The virulency of these two childish ailments has changed places.

One of the most important incidents that proved the value of the properly supervised school as an aid in preventing infections, came about during the wartime epidemic of influenza. There was a frightful sweep of the disease and there were not enough doctors or nurses to care for the cases nor enough undertakers to bury the dead. Theaters and moving-picture shows were closed by order of the Health Department which took charge. By their orders, also, all business had to function under a "stagger" system, certain groups of employees going to work at stated hours so that the subways, elevated railways and surface cars might not be overcrowded at any one time. The schools came in for their share of attention. All over the country schools were closed and the children allowed to play in the streets unsupervised and ready victims of the disease. One morning Commissioner Copeland sent for me. He told me that all public schools were to be closed at once. I do not know where I got the courage to remonstrate but youth gives one reckless strength of purpose. Anyway, I did protest and asked him a question:

"If you could have," I said, "a system where you could examine one fifth of the population of this city every morning and control every person who showed any symptom of influenza, what would it be worth to you?"

"Well, that would be almost priceless," he replied, "but we haven't got anything of the sort and why talk about it?"

"But of course we have," I said. "Won't you let me try out the idea I have in mind for a week or so? I want to see if I can't keep the six-to-fifteen-year age group in this city away from all danger of the 'flu.' I don't know that I can do it but I would awfully well like to have a chance."

"All right," he said, "I'll give you that chance but, remember, the responsibility is on your head." And as I was leaving the room, he casually added, "By the way, I am changing the name of German measles. Hereafter it will be known as 'Liberty measles'." And it did bear that extraordinary title for the duration of the war. War psychosis is a fearful and wonderful disrupter of horse sense.

But the schools were kept open. All of the inspectors and nurses were assigned solely to the care of this one disease. Every morning every school was visited by one of the doctors and the children were given a hurried inspection. The children went directly to their classrooms when they arrived at the school and directly home when the school was dismissed for the day. No class came into contact with any other class. So far as humanly possible, we watched those children. Not only were cases of influenza almost nonexistent among the children but the teachers kept well too. When the epidemic was over (incidentally, nothing more was said about closing the schools), we found that we had accomplished our purpose. The number of cases of influenza among children of school age was so small as to be negligible. There was no evidence at all, in this age group, that there had been any epidemic of influenza in the city. The number of children absent from school because of illness was lower than it had been for the same period the previous year. So far as I know, New York was the only large city that kept its schools open. That fact, and its results, received wide publicity and it was generally agreed that this method was the safe and sure one. It scored heavily for organized child hygiene work and was a great tribute to the doctors and nurses of the Bureau's staff.

When the great wave of propaganda for better teeth struck the United States, the Bureau of Child Hygiene plunged enthusiastically into the toothbrush war, of course. The incidence of bad teeth among the school children is so high that it baffles any corrective measures. We could not even try to fill one percent of the teeth that needed this care. Why not try to prevent tooth decay and have a campaign for clean mouths? We started in with all the enthusiasm of the convert. We installed a few dental clinics, staffed by dentists, for the more needy cases and we went in in a wholesale way for dental hygiene. Dr. Alfred C. Fones of Bridgeport, Connecticut, had started a training school for young women with the idea of teaching them the fundamentals of preventive dental care. Upon graduation, they were to be known as "dental hygienists" and were supposed to know all about how decay could be prevented so far as humanly possible. We took all of his graduates he could supply and soon afterward similar schools were opened in Boston, Rochester and in New York City. We established toothbrush drills in the classrooms. Any morning, a casual visitor to a school was apt to come upon an army of children all earnestly brushing their teeth. We spent a great deal of money on equipment and toothbrushes; we worked hard and long; we believed in the idea and certainly it was given every chance, but after years of trying to make toothbrushing a universal habit, we ended up just about where we began, which is only another way of saying that the results proved nothing at all and that part of our work was an absolute failure. Of course, the reason for our debacle is obvious. Dentists know more today about the reason for tooth decay than we did then. Keeping the teeth clean may be a hygienic habit just as washing the face is, but that the clean tooth does not decay is an exploded theory. We were, quite naturally, inundated with requests to use all kinds of dental cream and powder. We resisted them all and from the best inside information we could obtain, we invented our own dental powder which might be bought, in pound lots, for fifteen cents. It kept the teeth clean but it did not prevent decay. As selling propaganda, I can smile tolerantly at the claims made by manufacturers for their pastes and powders. Few of them are as honest as the firm which offered me six thousand dollars for my picture and a signed statement that merely said: "The sole function of a toothpaste is to clean the teeth. It has no medicinal properties whatever"; to be used for advertising, of course. I was quite willing to make the statement for the purpose of debunking the claims of grotesque advertising. But, upon consultation, I found that I was likely to be expelled from my various medical societies if I lent my name to any such purpose and I was not yet ready for this expulsion then. It does seem a pity that organized medicine can defeat its own purpose in so asinine a way. In all events they, meaning the manufacturers of dental pastes and powders, have gone back to their original fantastic claims. Someone may find out, some day, how dental decay may be easily prevented, but the great discoverer is not yet articulate.

But we had tried, and we tried again in the matter of bad eyesight, which is on the way to being the great American defect if one may judge by the number of people who wear glasses. We examined the children's eyes as nearly annually as we could. We fought for duller paper in textbooks, better spacing of the print and better classroom lighting in order to avoid eye-strain. But the incidence of defective eyesight is just as high as it ever was, possibly higher. I do think we got a note of sanity into the whole question of adenoids and enlarged and diseased tonsils, but there was little we could do with heart disease, besides establishing special classes for these children; and tuberculosis and orthopaedic defects seemed hopeless. We did manage to meet the challenge of undernourishment among these children. Here it was largely a matter of right feeding at regular hours, decent hygiene in the home and freedom from undue late hours and excitement. Public health education could go a long way along this road and we followed it with enthusiasm. It really meant altering the living habits of an entire population and that is a large order. But we did get results in the prevention of undernourishment even if they came slowly and were not spectacular. At any rate the proportion of cases showed a decline though it took an inordinate amount of work to bring this about.

Shortly before I retired, I found that a working lifetime of coping with this insanely complicated and probably hopeless matter of physical defects in school children was forcing me to make one last effort to find a way out. Again, I studied all the available facts, looking for an indicative pattern in them. Presently I began to think I saw some light. The New York Association for Improving the Condition of the Poor (another of those check-discouraging names) had some important figures, laid out in age groups, which were worth considering. They showed that the percentage of physical defects in children increased from 8.2 to 9.1 between six and eight years of age, rapidly declining thereafter to 1.7 at sixteen years. In order to check this and produce more detail, the Bureau rigidly examined 159,000 school children by age groups.

The results were more illuminating that I had hoped they could be. Sex had nothing to do with it. Both boys and girls had defects in the same proportion. And it was indubitably plain that the defects which we could hope to prevent or correct were present in largest force when the children were very young; that is, at the entering-school age of six years. Lung diseases, heart disease and nervous troubles stayed at about the same level throughout the groups at all ages, which probably meant that school life affected them not at all. Eye defects went up steadily until at the age of fourteen there were twice as many sufferers. Malnutrition, adenoids, enlarged and diseased tonsils and decayed teeth, all very popular difficulties, were at the height of their incidence at the entering-school age. It all resulted in a clear showing that if school health control was to evidence any symptom of sanity, most of our effort

should be spent on examining and securing treatment for
the child entering school for the first time. And so I made
the following statement in my printed report: "This study
seems to show that the expenditure of time and money to
make annual physical examinations of all school children
is unwarranted and unnecessary." I believed that then and
I believe it now. But the pressure was too great. I could
not induce the Health Department to make any such revolutionary change. They preferred the shapeless, pointless,
fragmentary round of haphazard examinations year after
year. Even today I go to meetings of school health authorities and hear the same old figures, the same old complaints,
the same old helplessness and the same old routine which
never made sense or produced any worth-while results and
which to me, today, sounds as archaic as an ox-cart.

It would have been even more revolutionary to follow
out the furthest implications of my figures and to try to
convince the powers that were that the only really sensible
thing to do would be to put the school child in the background, except for contagious diseases, and concentrate on
the pre-school child. For it is the neglected, unhappy, mis-
fit stepchild, known technically as "the pre-school child,"
who is our logical point of attack. Day nurseries and nursery schools touch only the surface of this problem, and
yet in it undoubtedly lies the solution of the health problem in schools. But I have been enough of a heretic in my
day to avoid any more such trouble in my resting years.
Perhaps, some day, the millennium will come. I can only
hope so.

People who write books about how much progress
human beings have made are always telling us that the
day of experimentation without a scientific background is
past. Working in the public health field is apt to make one

think twice about that dictum. No doubt the same is true of any other field where well established procedures make humans reluctant to reinspect their premises and contemplate change. In the days when I was trying to establish simple modification of whole milk, we used to have great arguments at the meetings of various medical societies. It was not because these doctors had found that my ideas were wrong; it was simply that they could not part from tradition. They had been told that certain procedures were correct and the simplest way was to continue them. In the face of my simple figures, they could only protest and deny. I had no scientific background for my proposed methods; they had plenty of what they thought was scientific background and they saw no reason to change their minds. And yet my whole-milk modification was a great success and is common practice today.

There was the time when I grew quite bothered about the open-air classrooms in the schools. Not that they were bad in themselves: far from it. They were almost too good. The difficulty seemed to be that there were too few of them and that they were set apart as a sort of shrine not to be approached by the common herd. Why, I pondered, should we limit the advantage of fresh air to a chosen few? Why should we select only the most tragic cases for life in the out-of-doors? Why should we breed more candidates for fresh-air classes than we could possibly accommodate?

In going about the schools, I was struck with the pale and anaemic appearance of the children kept in badly ventilated classrooms with closed windows and then contrasted their appearance with the twenty or thirty children who were in the one open-air classroom in the same building. Only the most undernourished children, the most anaemic and the most fragile children were considered candidates for the open-air class. Once established in it, their cheeks became redder, their appetites improved, they gained weight and made miraculous recoveries. It was all very dramatic but wholly wrong from the point of view of one who had to think in terms of the masses. Indoors, there would be too many small bodies, too closely contained in their clothes, perhaps not literally sewn in for the winter, but semi-permanently garbed just the same. The empty desks where children were absent with colds were numerous, the children's faces were pale, their eyes dull. Mine would have been the same way if I had had to stay in such a room six hours each day for five days each week. The Elizabeth McCormick Memorial Foundation in Chicago used to publish a poster which went to the heart of the matter, although I always suspected that much of the irony in it was by no means intended by the artist. It was a picture of a ragged, undersized, shivering boy looking up into the face of a healthy man standing outside of a door labelled "Open Air School." "Mister," he was saying, "how sick do I have to be to get in there?"

It was just one of those vague worries which you try to forget and which will persist in the back of your mind. One day, about that time, it became necessary for me to write a thesis for New York University in connection with my being awarded a degree of Dr.P.H. (Doctor of Public Health). The ventilation of school buildings was a thoroughly appropriate and not well explored subject. There were so many possible aspects of it that I narrowed my study down to *The Relation of Classroom Ventilation to Respiratory Diseases Among School Children.* Under the circumstances, the subject matter of the thesis had to be beyond challenge. With the aid of the New York Committee on Ventilation who kindly cooperated with me in checking up on all of the ventilating apparatus and temperatures, I worked on this for two years, and the results were highly interesting.

We selected groups of children of all racial types and social backgrounds and of related ages, carefully controlled, in rooms of three different classes: (a) those mechanically ventilated and kept at 68 degrees Fahrenheit; (b) those ventilated by open windows and kept at 50 degrees Fahrenheit (in these the children were supplied with warm clothing); and (c) classes ventilated by open windows with the heat kept at 68 degrees Fahrenheit. The results were unanswerable: the rate of absence from school on account of respiratory diseases (which means bronchitis and pneumonia) was 32 percent higher in the mechanically ventilated 68-degree rooms than in the open-window rooms kept at the same temperature, and 40 percent higher than in the open-window rooms kept at 50 degrees. In the mechanically ventilated, 68-degree classrooms the incidence of common colds was 98 percent higher than in open-window 68-degree rooms and about 70 percent higher than in the 50-degree rooms. That knowledge is just as useful in the home as it is in the school. And, when people objected that the cost of coal would be prohibitive in keeping rooms at 68 degrees with the windows open in zero weather, I had figures on that too, showing that the cost of the additional coal was no more than the depreciation and upkeep on a ventilating system, estimating that it would be replaced in twenty years. Much to my delight, this idea did seem productive of some good. Giving every child a chance at fresh air, instead of allowing only a picked few to have this privilege, attracted attention. A number of western cities built all of their new schools without any ventilating apparatus and relied solely on open window ventilation. At least two large private schools in New York City followed this example. But the New York City Public Schools continue to keep their windows closed and breed applicants for "Open-Air Classes."

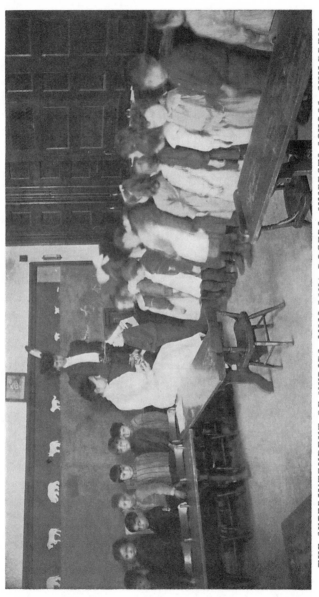

THE SUPERINTENDENT OF NURSES, MISS LINA ROGERS, INSPECTS SCHOOL CHILDREN

CHAPTER IX

IT MAY SEEM LIKE A COLD-BLOODED THING TO say, but someone ought to point out that the World War was a backhanded break for children—a break originating in the world's dismay at the appalling waste of human life, both at the front and behind the lines. As more and more thousands of men were slaughtered every day, the belligerent nations, on whatever side, began to see that new human lives, which could grow up to replace brutally extinguished adult lives, were extremely valuable national assets. When father had been torn apart by shrapnel or smothered by poison gas, his small sons and daughters, the parents of the future, took the spotlight as the hope of the nation. That is the handsomest way to put it. The ugliest way—and, I suspect, the truer—is to say flatly that it was the military usefulness of human life that wrought the change. When a nation is fighting a war or preparing for another, and the European nations have been doing one of those two things ever since 1914, it must look to its future supplies of cannon fodder. Particularly when supplies run short and unproductive militarism begins to lower the standard of living, rulers and governments begin to think hard about how best to conserve future citizens.

The child-conservation impulse was evidenced in America even before we entered the World War. In 1916 we had 8,914 cases of poliomyelitis, a disease that had been mildly epidemic on several previous occasions. But, to a world newly conscious of the importance of its children, the popular name for poliomyelitis, "infantile paralysis," conveyed an unbearable picture that, coupled with fear of infection, stirred up a mass emotion out of all proportion to the danger. Poliomyelitis had been made a reportable disease in 1910, but few cases had been reported and practically no precautions taken. It was not until this epidemic of 1916 that it was actually considered infectious. As a matter of fact the danger of infection was relatively slight. There were cases of infantile paralysis in 8,287 families, but 96 percent of these families had only one case. 16,500 children in these same families were intimately exposed to the infection and did not contract the disease. Nevertheless, it could be contracted, and the public accepted it as occasion for marked hysteria. General terror was fomented by the action taken by the New York City Department of Health and the resultant publicity. There were 21,603 cases of measles reported in 1916, 19,297 cases of tuberculosis, 13,521 cases of diphtheria—but the 8,900 children suffering from poliomyelitis formed the basis for a degree of panic that has never been equalled in the history of the New York City Health Department. All theatres, moving-picture houses, playgrounds and play streets were closed—all public gatherings prohibited. In September the opening of all schools was delayed for two weeks. The isolation period of all cases was extended to eight weeks. Large warning signs were placarded on the street walls of houses where cases occurred—even apartment houses were placarded at the main entrance as well as on the apartment-door of the afflicted family. There were even more startling rules: no child was allowed to leave the city or to enter it or to travel from one Borough to another, without an official certificate issued by the Department of Health stating that he lived in a house which had been free from polio-myelitis for at least two weeks. Hundreds of medical in-spectors and twenty-five officials from the United States Public Health Service were stationed at railroad stations, boat piers, ferry piers, and roads leading out of the city to enforce this regulation. The newspapers, of course, an-nounced these steps and treated them as the news they un-doubtedly were, and added their bit to the general air of catastrophe by publishing daily lists of cases, giving the name and address of each individual patient. Poliomyelitis is a serious and terrifying disease. It should receive all of the calm attention that is now being given it. But there should be no hysteria. The hope and promise of its preven-tion does not lie in the methods I have outlined; it lies in the orderly campaign that is now being waged. The first note of sanity was sounded in the establishment of the Warm Springs Foundation in Georgia, the second has come with the widespread interest shown in the President's Birthday Balls given throughout the country and now large groups of our citizens are giving largely of their interest and enthusiasm to make this one of our triumphs in the overcoming of disease.

I believe that the spreading war-psychology had some-thing to do with this over-dramatization. Nations already in the thick of actual war were more direct and reasonable in their efforts to preserve the younger generation. That point was made very clear to me shortly after the United States entered the war. I was walking down Fifth Avenue, already labelled "The Avenue of the Allies," on a bright spring day when all the flags were snapping and the uni-form on every other person I met looking handsomer than ever. Presently I met a woman I knew who was wearing a bright new khaki uniform, loaded down with all the leather and metal gadgets it would hold. She was sailing for London, she said, to supervise the work of feeding school-lunches to undernourished children in the London schools. Wasn't it horrible, she said, that on account of the war 12 percent of them were undernourished?

"That is horrible," I said, "but what would you say if I told you that, in New York, 21 percent of the school children are undernourished, and largely on account of that same war?"

I was not trying to stop her from going to London. Perhaps it was my own lack of a uniform that made me so sharp about it. For I never got to France and I never buttoned a khaki coat around myself, even though I held a high military rank. I have never been able to understand just why the office of the Surgeon-General of the United States proceeded as it did in my case. Almost as soon as the United States declared war, a large international organization asked me to give up my New York post and go to France to take charge of all its work with refugee and homeless children. A huge and important and intoxicatingly useful job which I accepted with joy. And then, not twenty-four hours later, a telegram came from Washington. The powers there knew all about my offer—and disapproved. I was needed at home more than in France, they said, when I went to Washington to see about it. I would be good enough to tell these people that I had changed my mind and give no reason for my refusal.

It was a desperate position to force anybody into, for it made me look both impolite and yellow, which is not a palatable combination. But it had to be done, so I did it, and trailed back to pick up the exacting routine of the Bureau of Child Hygiene again. Presently I received a confidential communication from the office of the Surgeon-General of the United States Public Health Service: an elaborately engraved certificate informing me I had been appointed an Assistant Surgeon-General with the rank of Major in this branch of our government. I liked that, all the more because I am pretty sure I was the first woman ever to receive so high-ranking a commission. But I would have felt a good deal better about the whole thing if that envelope had instead contained permission for me to go to France in almost any capacity.

My statement that 21 percent of New York's school children were undernourished was no exaggeration. War prices were largely responsible. The war boom had raised prices to high points, for one thing, and for another, so much of the teeming American supply of various food-stuffs was being shipped to Europe that, although there was enough to keep all from starving, the markets seldom had a chance to level off with increases in available supplies. So, all through the war, we had to add a widespread malnutrition program to our already overloaded schedules. We fed the children lunches; we campaigned to get each child an extra spoonful of oil, even if butter was economically out of the question; we fought to conserve the milk supply so as to divert more of it to children's use. It was a long hard pull but, by the time the war was over, the percentage of undernourishment among New York children was almost as low as that in London and we could tell ourselves that, in general, we were looking after our own children almost as well as if they had been poor little Belgians. It was during this period that I coined a rhetorical contrast which, I think, made more people think about child welfare than anything else I ever said or wrote: the simple statement that "It's six times safer to be a soldier in the trenches of France than to be born a baby in the United States."

Long after the war was over, the American people kept on with this queer insistence on doing better by one's neighbors' children than by one's own. It will be remembered how large a part children played in the advertisement of American post-war relief activities. The starving Belgian and Armenian and, immediately after the war, starving Russian and German and Austrian children appealed far more successfully to the American pocketbook than the equally miserable and rickety little people on Washington Street, Manhattan Island. Yet I should not be too disturbed about that, I suppose. It was a long time happening, but eventually it was true that all this agitation about other people's small unfortunates produced a psychological effect which made things much better for the American child. Although the New York Bureau of Child Hygiene had had plenty of publicity before the war, its example had been followed in only five states by 1914. During and after the war the landslide began, however. State after state wanted to start a Bureau of Child Hygiene. City after city was inspired with the same hope, and in each case someone was sent to my office to "see how it could be done." The idea was growing. It was to grow still more rapidly later and I could see the day in the future when it would pervade the country. I think it was about this time that I made up my mind that my term of office should be limited by this growth. I promised myself that when the forty-eighth state should have organized a Bureau of Child Hygiene, I would retire. By 1923 all forty-eight states had such bureaus, and I kept my promise. It is a rare privilege to have been present at the birth of a great and new idea and see it grow to maturity, even though some of its growth must be credited to a world disaster.

America furnished not only most of the supplies for the European children, but also a great deal of the technical experience for the people in charge. Almost as soon as the war began to look like a long and serious business, dignitaries came flocking from Europe to New York to find out how New York's Bureau of Child Hygiene worked and how much of its procedure was applicable to their problem. From all countries on both sides—enthusiastic Frenchmen; peering, solemn and intelligent Germans; voluble Russians; close-mouthed and sharp-eyed Englishmen; smiling delegations from China and Japan. It was extraordinarily flattering. We knew, of course, that our Bureau was the only one of its kind in the world, but we had not realized that it had become internationally famous. We showed them everything and went far out of our way to work out answers to their different problems and then back they went to report and set up organizations.

But the more I thought it over, the more disturbed I became. Our heart-warming progress in revolutionizing child care had been possible only because the American public had learned to consider it intolerable that babies and children should die needlessly or grow up needlessly handicapped. But it had taken the sinister stimulus of mass-murder to make the fighting nations see the necessity for saving children. The French had anticipated some of our developments years before the Bureau of Child Hygiene was founded; baby health stations, for instance. But they did nothing on any large scale with the idea until the piling up of corpses in the trenches of the western front forced them to speculate, subconsciously perhaps, as to how many recruits would be available for conscription in 1939.

The various European dictatorships, red and black alike, are still carrying on that tradition, probably for the same uncomfortable reason. Only a few years ago I met at dinner a certain foreign dignitary high in power in a famous dictatorship. When he had the opportunity he spoke to me, and reminded me that he and I had met during the war, when he was on a special mission to the United States.

"You must remember," he said, "that I asked you to draw up a scheme for child welfare in my country. You spent two or three weeks doing it in great detail." I asked how the scheme had worked out. "Very well," he said, "and especially well for me. They neglected it until recently; but then one day the Chief suddenly summoned me"—he didn't say Chief, but I'd rather not use the word that would make it possible to identify him—"and told me that he wanted me to draw up plans for a national child welfare scheme, at once. So I went back to my office and got out of my file the copy of your plan almost twenty years old, had it translated and sent to the Chief as my own work and," he said, patting himself on a particularly gorgeous medal, "this is what I got for it."

Such grim general considerations did not, however, keep me from realizing that these inquisitive visitors were fine people almost without exception, as they should have been in that kind of work. There were dozens of them coming day after day not only during these years but all through the years both before and after the war. Dr. Armand de Lille and Dr. René Sand, the French and Belgian inquirers respectively, were a joy to meet. The English contingent, numerous and highly pleasant, were all titled somehow, no doubt on the principle that there was nothing like a handle to your name for making a good impression on those

Americans. The Duchess of Marlborough, a very simple, charming person, came over to buy equipment for a new English children's hospital. I helped her plan out what she needed and showed her where to buy it. Lady Aberdeen made several trips on one and another kind of war-work. She was a grand person. Her husband, an extremely august old gentleman who was then Lord-Lieutenant of Ireland, if I remember correctly, and had been Governor-General of Canada, was even more certain of that than I was. He accompanied her on one of her trips and always sat on the platform behind her when she was making a speech. Lady Aberdeen was an excellent speaker and, every time she scored a hit, Lord Aberdeen would thump on the crown of his silk topper which he held decorously between his knees, tomtom-fashion, and give tongue as if he had been in the House of Lords: "Hear, hear! . . . Hear, hear!" Only, since he pronounced it in true parliamentary fashion: "Hyah, hyah!" I doubt if a good half of the audience had any notion of what this peculiar English custom of saying "Yah, yah!" in the middle of a speech was all about.

The late Sir Leslie MacKenzie, Sir Arthur Newsholme and the late Sir George Newman were other charming and competent English welfare people who came to see us. Sir George was then Medical Officer of Health in the English Health Ministry. I spent many days in the field with him examining minutely the various branches of the New York City Bureau of Child Hygiene. In the end he tried to persuade me to go back to London with him where he said he could guarantee me the position of Health Director for the whole London school system. It was a tempting offer. I have always been fond of the English and possess more respect for their ways of doing things than Americans are supposed to have. But something Sir George himself had said when he was going through our own New York schools with me had already shown me why I would have to refuse this offer. We were talking with the principal of an East Side school of some 2,000 girls. At that time immigration was still at a high flow. Sir George expressed surprise at the fact that they all spoke quite good English. Weren't New York school-children in the poorer districts largely immigrants' children? Or were this lot all born in New York?

"Oh, no," said the principal, "very few. Practically all born abroad, I should say."

"Good heavens!" said Sir George. "How do you people do this sort of thing? We've no problem to match it at all. In Berlin the poor are German, are thoroughly fitted for the German environment. In London, they are all English and fitted to be Englishmen. But here—you have the poor of every country on earth to contend with. It's deeply impressive, I assure you."

So it struck me that, by the same token, a New Yorker would be most ill advised to try to fit herself into an English situation. I was, after all, doing the same work in New York, and it was still urgent and important. I wondered whether we would welcome an Englishman at the head of our school health work. Such jobs abroad, I decided, belonged to citizens or subjects of the countries concerned. I would lay out programs, give advice, work myself hard to show these people what we did and why. But I should never have been able to be happy as an expatriate expert.

This going about with distinguished visitors was by no means all hard work and no play. There was the occasion when Sir George Newman and Lord Astor (they sent us the one available Lord with an American background) and another knight whose name I cannot remember, and I were all ejected from one of Lord Astor's apartments. It was a fine bit of farce all the way through. When I started to commandeer a Health Department car to use for this particular party, the best I could get was a ramshackle, dusty touring-car, with a chauffeur who had neglected to put on a collar. It looked disreputable enough when I drove up in it to the Waldorf-Astoria. It looked even more so when this peer of the realm and his two knight-companions came out and got into it. Not because it looked unworthy of them. On the contrary, to American eyes it looked a little better than they did. I was aware that Englishmen traditionally wore baggy tweeds, but I had not been aware that any tweeds could be that baggy or that cloth caps, the kind corner-loafers wear, were part of the outfit too.

We worked hard all day, visiting baby clinics and schools. We had stopped at a cafeteria in the Bronx, all of us bringing our food to the same table and cheerily lunching with the chauffeur, who steadily rebuffed these queer strangers' efforts to engage him in conversation. It was a hot, steamy day in early summer and every ten minutes we grew dustier, stickier and seedier to the dispassionate eye. Then, as we started home, Lord Astor said that since the American type of large, expensive apartment house was non-existent in London in those days, he wanted to show one to these Englishmen.

"I own an apartment house called the Apthorp down here," he said. "May we drop in there?"

So we dropped in at the Apthorp, on upper Broadway, an impressive kind of apartment house with a smart and very dapper West Indian hall boy, one of those sing-song and rather severe West Indians. When we entered, he sized us up as either hoboes or swindlers—so much was obvious. When Lord Astor said he wanted to show these friends of his one of the apartments, the boy froze like a dowager with her train stepped on.

"We've nothing to show you," he said, ice clinking in his voice.

"Now come," said Lord Astor, "I happen to know there are some vacancies. We must go up at once. We're in a hurry."

"Look here," said the boy, "you'd better go along quietly. I don't want to have to make trouble for you."

"But," said Lord Astor, "I'm Lord Astor. I own this building."

"*Will* you get out of here before I call the police?" said the boy.

So we got out of there, with the boy following us to see we didn't steal a statue on the way out. Then, being a smart lad, as I said, he managed to read the golden letters "H.D." beneath the grime and mud on the door of our disreputable car. He asked the chauffeur a few questions and then, turning dusky purple, began to apologize just as the driver let in the clutch. As we rattled away, we all looked at one another and began to laugh.

"What are you going to do about the hall boy?" I asked, as soon as I got my breath back.

Lord Astor looked at himself and then at the others.

"Nothing whatever," he said. "He was quite right. If he had let us in, I'd have had him discharged."

That combination of a car, a celebrity and a tour of child-welfare facilities often provided some amusement. Once I had recovered from its effects, I knew I had had a very fine time as escort for a similar tour with Theodore Roosevelt. That day combined in a nut-shell all the excitement, the hurry and the feverishness of the period.

It was fairly early in 1918, as I remember. It was

Colonel Roosevelt's idea to begin with, starting with a telephone message from his secretary indicating that the Colonel had developed a lively interest in the Bureau's work and wouldn't we like to take him around and show him what we were doing? The answer was obviously yes. An appointment was made. I suspected it was going to be quite a day, so, for moral support, I drafted Dr. Henry Dwight Chapin as my companion, and up we went to the Colonel's office to escort him on the rounds. Our only special preparations consisted of using the Department of Health's best-looking car as a tribute to the Colonel's dignity, and asking the Police Department to detail a few men to the places we were to visit—in case of crowds. The Colonel drew a crowd wherever he went. When it came to attracting public attention, he was a kind of human three-alarm fire.

The fun began the moment we were ushered into the Colonel's office. He squared round and faced us immediately—the angriest man I ever saw in my life, I think: mustache bristling, eyes glowing behind his thick-lensed glasses and voice telling us just what he thought of us.

"I'm not going with you at all," he told us. "I wanted this trip to be quiet and unmolested—above all I wanted to avoid any publicity—and yet you've gone ahead and had it announced in the papers—"

I protested that we had done no such thing. I had not said a word about it to a reporter or to anyone connected with journalism and, so far as I knew, there had been no publicity at all.

"Oh, there hasn't?" he roared, bouncing out of his chair. "I'm through with you and the whole thing. I resent this whole business and I refuse to make myself a party to it by going out with you." Then he shouted for his secretary to bring him the morning paper and began wading through it, snorting and growling like one of his own western grizzly bears. It took a long time to find the item, but in the end he turned up a tiny paragraph at the foot of a column on one of the back pages about how Colonel Roosevelt was planning to visit baby health stations that morning. I tried to explain that perhaps my request for police details had enabled a police reporter to pick it up. But he would listen to no explanations.

When we started to leave after his tenth repetition of "I'm disgusted with the whole thing and I'm not going with you," he suddenly became relatively friendly. "Either of you in a hurry?" he asked. When we said why, no, in some surprise and sat down again, he leaned forward and asked: "Look here, what do you think of the way this war's being managed?" Dr. Chapin and I sputtered something feeble, but it did not matter what we said because the Colonel was distinctly not listening. Instead he was warming up to the first few sentences of a sizzling speech. "I'll tell you what I think of this war," he began and, for the next half hour, he never stopped to draw breath. We just sat there, speechless, swamped under a brilliant oratorical outpouring of scorn and anger. He told us exactly where President Wilson was wrong and exactly why Theodore Roosevelt should have been given a large hand in the management of the war and exactly what he would do if he were in the saddle and why anything else was tragic, idiotic, bungling, treacherous, unforgivable nonsense. It really was inspiring to hear him—beyond any question the best speech I had heard the Colonel make in twenty years of listening to him.

It evidently did him good to state his opinions so fully,

so forcibly and so frankly. When he had finished and the whole administration was figuratively lying about the office in shreds and tatters, he leaned back in his chair, grinned at us with amiable ferocity and said:

"Well, I don't want to disappoint you. Maybe I will go with you after all. Let's make it day after tomorrow—and remember, no publicity." We swore there would be no publicity. When he called in his secretary to have her make a note of the engagement, she was solemnly instructed to make every effort to keep the expedition out of the papers. As we were leaving, he turned again to the secretary: "Well, I don't know," he said, "the newspaper boys are good fellows and it might make nice copy for them— maybe you'd better call up the *Sun* and the Associated Press and see if they'd like to send somebody along with us on Thursday." Then, turning to me: "Perhaps we could wind up some place where there's an auditorium," he said. "Then we could—yes—" to the secretary—"call up all the newspapers and tell them I'll make a speech to all the reporters they want to send."

That was the way he went about avoiding publicity. Even so, not wanting to speak out of turn, I stuck to my end of the bargain and gave the press no notice from the Bureau, merely asked the Police Commissioner to supply plenty of police coverage at all the stops we were planning to make. Within a few hours Health Department doctors and nurses who had heard the news by grapevine telegraph were coming in to ask me if they could be on duty at the first baby health station we were to visit so they could see the Colonel.

Being nervous about managing what was turning into a traveling circus, I left it to Dr. Chapin to go for the

Colonel on Thursday morning and went myself to the first stop of the itinerary to see that all was ready. The front room was crowded with mothers and babies and the back room full of doctors and nurses thrilled over the approaching great man. He arrived in style, in the big shiny department car, followed by a string of a dozen or fifteen taxis packed full of reporters, news-photographers and newsreel cameramen with all their equipment, the whole cavalcade roaring through the narrow East Side streets with the air of a royal procession in a hurry. Naturally there was a first-class crowd for the photographers to work on. The moment the Colonel stepped out of the car he pounced on a policeman and began shaking him by the hand: "I know you," he said. "I appointed you to the force back when I was Police Commissioner, didn't I?" And he and this policeman proceeded to have an Old Home Week there on the sidewalk, with news-cameras clicking merrily, until I tore them apart and got the Colonel inside.

Considering that so much of the medical and nursing staff of the Bureau was wasting its morning in the back room, I immediately asked the Colonel if he would mind stepping in and saying "Hello" to them. When I got him inside, I found he expected to be personally introduced to each of them. They were all members of my Bureau, but names have always been one of my major stumbling-blocks and, as I took the Colonel around, I asked to have one of my supervisors at my elbow so he might whisper their names in my ear. That made it all the more dramatic when, as we were leaving, the Colonel said he wanted to say goodbye all around—and, although I can still hardly believe it, he actually went back and shook hands with every one of those people all over again and called each one of thirty-odd perfect strangers *by name*. If I had seen that done on the vaudeville stage, I should have called it a trick.

That started us off in fine style. All the rest of the day we went rushing around New York, stopping at various Bureau stations, schools and institutions for children, going in to let the Colonel talk to the mothers and children and tell them about his own grandchildren. Every time we came out of a station or a school we would have our pictures taken again, the Colonel standing between Dr. Chapin and me, and grinning so refulgently that the cameramen must have had to stop down their lenses. I think we had our pictures taken on an average of every fifteen minutes for six hours. But between times he plied me with the shrewdest and best informed set of questions I ever listened to. At five o'clock we reached the Post-Graduate Hospital where Dr. Chapin had arranged for the use of the auditorium. I was a little afraid that once the Colonel got on his feet he would be unable to resist the temptation to repeat his violent dissertation on the way the war was being handled; but no, he stood up and made a speech brimming over with intelligent eulogy of child welfare work. It was old stuff to the assembled press, but it had all been new and glorious to him and he said so as emphatically and at as much length as if the entire Bureau of Child Hygiene had been his own baby.

I was exhausted by that time—so were Dr. Chapin and the reporters and photographers. But, when we climbed wearily back into the car for the last time and asked the Colonel if he wanted us to take him home: "No," he said, "not home. Drop me at the Union League Club. I'll be dressing there before I go on to a dinner where I have to make a speech." Well, after all, he was the man who coined the phrase "the strenuous life." He was apparently quite capable of going through the whole performance again without stopping for breath. We left him at the club and went home to try to recuperate.

Yes, odd events happened in those queerly kinetic years. I had the privilege, shared with a great many other women, of being suspected of mildly radical sympathies which during the war were, of course, synonymous with giving aid and comfort to the enemy. I was no pacifist whatever. I would hardly have received that major's commission if I had been. But I did belong to a luncheon club for women active in various social and economic movements, and that was apparently enough. The name of the club was, and still is, Heterodoxy. Perhaps it was the name that alarmed the spy-chasers. Perhaps it was true, as legend said, that a worried member of Heterodoxy had written a letter calling on the secret service men to keep an eye on the club's weekly meetings because its rolls contained so many pacifists and radicals. The fantastic result was that we really did have to shift our meeting-place every week to keep from being watched. It was just like an E. Phillips Oppenheim novel. All except the characters, that is. My colleagues in treason were not sloe-eyed countesses with small pearl-handled revolvers in their pocketbooks but people like Crystal Eastman, Fannie Hurst, Rose Pastor Stokes, Inez Haynes Irwin, Fola La Follette and Mabel Dodge Luhan.

We had Amy Lowell to address a meeting once, I remember. She dealt very pleasantly with her theories of poetry and such general subjects and then asked if anybody would like her to read some of her poems. That produced a landslide of requests. Member after member demanded a special favorite, and each selection was more sentimental than the last, which had dripped with sweet sorrows of one sort or another. It was all so sad that Rose

Pastor Stokes turned around and laid her head on her neighbor's shoulder and cried down her neck, sobbing an obbligato to Miss Lowell's sonorous voice. The poetess stood it as long as she could and then:

"I'm through," she said. "They told me I was to be speaking to a group of intellectual, realistic, tough-minded leaders in the women's world. Instead I find a group that wants nothing but my most sentimental things. Good afternoon!" And she poked her cigar into her mouth and walked out glowering.

It may have been my connection with Heterodoxy that offended the Daughters of the American Revolution. Or perhaps it was my connection with the Federal Children's Bureau, which, for some reason or other, struck the stupider kind of conservatives as vaguely subversive when it was first started. I did not know I was on the D. A. R. blacklist until I received an invitation from a committee, headed by Heywood Broun, for a dinner given by and for all people who were not to be allowed to address meetings of the D. A. R., wherever found. I went to the dinner and had a very fine time in the very best of company—that list was the cream of American intellectuals with a slightly liberal leaning, for it was at the time when the Red-hunt was at its hottest.

I enjoyed it all the more in remembering that not long before I had been a Daughter of the American Revolution myself. A patient of mine insisted that I should join the D. A. R.—surely a woman with my fine old American background could raise a revolutionary ancestor. Finally she went so far as to say that, if I didn't join the D. A. R. she might have to look for another doctor. That was serious, so I checked up on my forebears, discovered that a good half dozen of my ancestors had fought the British,

and duly joined. Not long afterward, however, my patient
died. The dues were not high, but they struck me as absolutely wasted money, so I immediately resigned.

Until I received that dinner invitation, I never regretted
it. Then, however, I saw what a blunder I had committed.
It would have been much better if the D. A. R. had black-
listed me while I was still on their membership-roll.

There was any amount of confusion, during the war
years, about the precise point where liberalism lapsed into
dangerous radicalism. I belonged to one organization in
the early years of the war, before we entered the holocaust,
that I look back upon with awe and a vague feeling of
nostalgia. The air was full of public-spirited efforts of one
sort or another at that time, but in this case a full-fledged
idealist was found in a strictly scientific laboratory: the
late Dr. S. J. Meltzer. He was an important official in the
Rockefeller Institute, and when the war began in Europe
he had the idea that all doctors were above factional strife
and feelings. He planned and put into operation an organization called "The War Brotherhood," the membership of
which was to be made up of all doctors from all nations at
war. In the light of what happened afterwards and what is
happening today, Dr. Meltzer's ideals now seem curiously
eccentric. But they did not seem so then. Among the doctors in the United States, the idea attracted the very best:
the list of members sounds like an honor roll of American
medicine. We had many meetings all permeated with our
high purpose. We proposed to keep doctors neutral. It
never occurred to us that this was an impossible task.
Europe did not take kindly to our offer of brotherhood. It
became apparent almost at once that doctors are as human
and as nationalistic as anyone else. We still had hopes of
our own, but later, when we entered the war, American

doctors became as partisan as the others, and the Brotherhood dissolved.

That organization is now merely a bit of Americana from the pre-war period. As I was the only woman to hold office in the War Brotherhood, it marked my idealistic contribution to a world that has long since departed. It is hard now to remember that it ever existed.

When the Bureau of Child Hygiene was fairly started on its career, we fell heir to one of the neglected stepchildren of the Department. This was the issuance of employment certificates to children allowing them to leave school and go to work. While this would seem to be a matter belonging wholly to the jurisdiction of the Board of Education, the Legislature, in its wisdom, had handed the enforcement of this law to the Department of Health because a physical examination was to be made of each child and the granting, or with-holding, of the certificate depended upon the physical condition of the child.

We soon found that these presumed physical examinations were a farce and that very little political pressure was needed to assure any child, no matter how underweight or physically handicapped he might be, of getting his certificate without any difficulty. It was an intrenched racket. The law at that time required a child to be fourteen years old and to have completed the eighth grade of school work. The enforcement was so lax that practically any child with a very little dressing of his age could get a certificate at any time. To give a little idea of how lax this enforcement was, I remember my first contact with the office force in the Department assigned to this duty. I wandered into the office one day and on the scales stood a child, palpably not much over ten years old, peaked and thin and with his pockets protruding in knobby excresences that looked like huge swellings at various parts of his anatomy. The recorded weight was all right for a boy of fourteen and his school record looked all right also. But as he stepped down from the scales, I called him to me. "Let's see what you have in your pockets?" I queried. Quite calmly he began to disgorge the lumps and the net result was over twenty pounds of lead which he had spread over his person to get his weight up to the required degree. Anyone could have noticed it but no one did. Anyway, our clean-up began at once.

It was a long and difficult task to restore some sanity to this branch of our work and to get the system in a condition so that the children might be protected so far as the law allowed. The New York State Child Labor Committee came to my aid. Miss Jeannie Minor of that Committee came to work with me as the head of that division of our work and with the aid of Mr. George A. Hall, who is still the Committee's Secretary, we gradually got the work in such good condition that for many years it ranked first in the State in the enforcement of the law and in the protection of the child. But, try as we would, it all seemed rather futile to me. Why should children work? What sort of country was this that had to subsist, in part at least, upon the toil and labor of the young? It was easy enough to see that the fault was basic and that no amount of careful work in our office did anything more than help enforce a bad law. And so, I became an ardent worker in the attempt to get a Federal Amendment prohibiting all child labor in the United States. That was thirty years ago and I am still working for the same end.

We have made some progress, due largely I think to the adult need of the jobs that children used to get with little or no trouble. Slowly, but surely, various states have passed adequate laws prohibiting child labor, but the Federal Amendment, passed by Congress in 1924, still hangs fire. The age at which these certificates may be issued has gradually been raised to sixteen, in many states, but there are still too many states which allow little children to work long hours for little pay. The big ray of hope has come recently. The Fair Labor Standards Act of 1938 bans interstate commerce in articles made wholly, or in part, by children under sixteen years of age.

I can think of no potent arguments in favor of child labor. It is a shameful and degrading thing that childhood should lose the essence of its being so that the men who employ these children may live at ease. States rights can become a sad failure when they are invoked to perpetuate such an evil. We are, on the whole, a decent and warmhearted people who love our children. Can't we forget political animosities and get together to give these thousands of children the protection from exploitation that we want for our own children? Can't we at last abolish all child labor, in this country, for all time?

CHAPTER X

Up to 1914 I THINK I COULD CONSCIENTIOUSLY
have testified on oath that, in my opinion, I was leading
a fairly active life. The foregoing pages merely summarize
and actually give very little idea of the amount of skirmish-
ing about, plus omnipresent, desk-confining detail, that
goes into the organization and management of an under-
taking like the Bureau of Child Hygiene. During the next
five or six years, however, I began to look back on the
pre-war period as a period of dignified relaxation. And I
am not speaking merely of the war. Everything started
whirling at once that year; why I do not know. Suffrage,
for instance. Once I start talking suffrage and the general
crisis in the cause of women's rights with which the height
of American suffrage agitation coincided, I indulge in another period of marveling at the difference twenty years
has made.

In the spring of 1914 I received a letter from the Philadelphia College of Physicians asking me to read a paper
before them on some aspect of my child health work. I assumed that the Philadelphia College of Physicians was
about the same as the New York Academy of Medicine, an
institution with which I have had many contacts, both
friendly and otherwise. When I reached Philadelphia,
however, there was a note waiting for me at my hotel asking me to dine with twelve of the College doctors at the
Union League. I was the only woman in the clubhouse.

From the way the place felt and the way the members' faces froze into paralytic astonishment as I passed, I suspect I was the only woman who ever *had* been in the clubhouse. The dinner was a highly formal, extremely enjoyable, but definitely stately occasion. I could not understand why they were making so much social fuss over the mere reading of a paper before a first-rate medical society, or why I had been honored with this exclusively male society.

After dinner, my twelve hosts formed up in a column and escorted me in an impressive procession of motor cars to the College itself. There were no women in the audience there either. Then the President of the college rose to introduce me to this solemn assemblage of medical men, and they *were* an impressive-looking group.

"Gentlemen," he said, "this is a remarkable occasion. For the first time since the Philadelphia College of Physicians was founded in 1787, a woman has been allowed to enter its premises." I learned privately afterwards that it was only after months of debate that the College had decided to invite me at all.

That was more than half a century after Dr. Blackwell had started women in medical practice in America. The name of Pankhurst was already a household word wherever newspapers were read and periodicals of all kinds had been talking about the New Woman for thirty years. But that is not to be taken as evidence of peculiar conservatism, in Philadelphia. I was presently to encounter a less gentlemanly version of the same tradition among medical students at the New York University-Bellevue Hospital Medical School in my own New York.

There were several absurdities about that incident. It all began when Dr. William H. Park, who was both dean of the N. Y. U. medical school and laboratory-director in the

New York Department of Health, asked me to lecture on
child hygiene in a new course the school was giving to
lead up to the new degree of Doctor of Public Health. I
reflected that presently I would be taking into the Bureau
new men who could write Dr.P.H. after their names,
whereas I would be without that extremely pertinent degree. So, in the interests of discipline, I offered Dr. Park a
bargain : I would give those lectures on child hygiene at
Bellevue if he would let me enroll in the course myself, so
I could take a Dr.P.H. degree too. He refused. The idea of
letting me take the same course in which I was lecturing
was not what bothered him. It was the college regulations
forbidding women in any courses whatever. I can hardly
be accused of acting unreasonably because I declined to act
as teacher in an institution that considered me unfit for
instruction.

Dr. Park tried for some time to find someone to lecture
in that part of the course. No one would. Child hygiene
was not as well known a subject then as it has since become.
So he returned to me and again I refused except on that
one condition and the argument went back and forth until
we were all heartily sick of it. Finally the college surren-
dered. I was to be allowed to take the two-year course in
public health and get my degree. Naturally they could not
admit me and deny entrance to other women, so another
set of long-barred doors opened to the female of the species.

With that farcical beginning, I lectured to Bellevue
students for fifteen years. They never allowed me to forget that I was the first woman ever to impose herself on
the college. Their method of keeping me reminded derived
directly from my first lecture, which was a nerve-racking
occasion. I stood down in a well with tiers of seats rising
all around me, surgical-theater fashion, and the seats were

filled with unruly, impatient, hardboiled young men. I looked them over and opened my mouth to begin the lecture. Instantly, before a syllable could be heard, they began to clap—thunderously, deafeningly, grinning and pounding their palms together. Then the only possible way of saving my face occurred to me. I threw back my head and roared with laughter, laughing at them and with them at the same time—and they stopped, as if somebody had turned a switch. I began to lecture like mad before they changed their minds, and they heard me in dead silence to the end. But, the moment I stopped speaking at the end of the hour, that horrible clapping began again. Frightened and tired as I was from talking a solid hour against a gloweringly hostile audience, I fled at top speed. Every lecture I gave at Bellevue, from 1915 through to 1930, was clapped in and clapped out that way; not the spontaneous burst of real applause that can sound so heart-warming, but instead the flat, contemptuous whacking rhythms with which the crowd at a baseball game walk an unpopular player in from the outfield.

By that time I was in the middle of the suffrage fight, as I should have been as a conspicuous woman in government service. I have explained before that I did not start out as a feminist at all. But it was impossible to resist the psychological suction which gradually drew you into active participation in the great struggle to get political recognition of the fact that women are as much human beings as men are. Fundamentally that was what we were all after. We suffrage agitators talked a great deal about how women's votes would clean up political corruption and encourage legislation and discourage wars, high-sounding hopes which seemed plausible enough at the time. But most of that was no more than strategic special pleading before the court of public opinion. Deep down what held us together was our sense of how unfair and absurd it was that the male half of the world should possess responsibilities from which we were excluded.

My early indifference to the suffrage issue broke down soon enough for me to be one of the five or six original members of the College Equal Suffrage League, an organization of college women working for the vote. We tried particularly to emphasize the absurdities of denying to well-educated women a privilege accorded to semi-illiterate men. When the League was founded, there were only half a dozen women college graduates who dared belong to such an association. When asked to become a member, the average college woman acted as if you had suggested she play Lady Godiva at a stag-picnic. But that only goes to show the pathetically small scale of the suffrage movement within a few years of its great triumph.

The annual suffrage parade up Fifth Avenue, for instance, which eventually became one of the most impressive shows in American life, had only five hundred marchers the first time it braved public scorn. I was one of the five hundred, all of us about as excited and apprehensive as if we had been early Christian martyrs lining up for the grand march into the Colosseum. When I heard the command to march, I was literally not at all sure that the nerves and muscles in my quivering legs would meet their assignment. None of us had any idea how the public would react to the idea of a group of women making a public show of themselves, and that was pretty certainly the way the man in the street was going to look at it those days. So our orders were to march straight ahead, eyes front, no matter what happened.

A group of some fifty courageous men, headed by Oswald Garrison Villard, marched with us and carried banners and placards boosting our cause as fervidly as we were boosting it ourselves. When this men's section swung into line and stepped out into Fifth Avenue, we all heard a roar of laughter go up and pursue them like a vanishing wave. Here it comes, we thought, glancing out of the corners of our eyes at the grinning, sniggering crowd. But they had a respectable reason for their mirth. Somebody had been in too much of a hurry handing out the placards, and one of the men, striding along conspicuously in the van of the men's section, was carrying a large sign that read: "Men can vote—why can't we?"

When we got that away from him, the spectators quieted down somewhat. There was plenty of jeering, but there was also a fair amount of encouragement for us. The chief danger was from the sheer bulk of the crowd. Police protection was most inadequate and presently the spectators were pressing inquisitively in from the sidewalks, as crowds always will when there is nothing to hold them back, threatening to smother the parade without trying to. But we stepped right ahead, chins up and out, and our immediate path was kept clear by a kind of psychological right of eminent domain.

Every year after that experiment, the suffrage parade was bigger, more impressive and more picturesque, and every year we drew larger and more friendly crowds. Different units in the parade had special costuming both to work up morale among their members and to increase the spectacular aspects of the show; we college women, for instance, did our parading as a solid phalanx of academic caps and gowns—and there were masses of brilliant scarves and magnificent women-riders dashing up and down on horseback, acting as marshals and incidentally demonstrating to the crowd that a female creature, for all this weaker sex talk, could sit a horse like a cavalry colonel. The spectacle of Inez Milholland, the beautiful Joan of Arc of the suffrage movement, wearing a long, snow-white riding habit and clattering up and down on a white horse, was probably worth thousands of votes to us. The whole thing was a grand show in the bright sunshine of early fall when the parade was usually held; the air just a little crisp, the bands playing and thousands on thousands of determined and disciplined women steadily marching from Union Square to 59th Street in a demonstration of solidarity that made each individual in the line of march feel like a giantess in her own right. What a thrill we did get out of it! I am not much of a walker, but every time we got to the Plaza and were ordered to disband, I felt childishly disappointed because we could not go right back to Union Square and start over again.

The first few years police protection was consistently bad: a few patrolmen scattered along, but evidently under no orders to do anything about the crowd's tendency to ooze into the street and swamp us. It was so bad that there was every reason to suspect the city authorities of purposely neglecting their responsibilities in hope that the parade would be broken up. Every year there was a bigger quarrel between the suffrage leaders and the city on this point, until finally the city was shamed into assigning plenty of men in uniform with strict orders to keep the crowd back. The policemen loved it. When we were stopped to let cross-traffic through, they would saunter over and tell us they were all for us and we were doing a fine thing. Commend me to policemen. I have had a good deal of experience with them and, give them half a chance, they are always a good lot.

We might have had less pleasant experiences if we had fought our battle along the militant lines favored by Mrs. Pankhurst's followers in England, where suffragettes raided the House of Commons, chained themselves to railings, threw stones, went on hunger-strikes after being thrown into jail, and generally had a violent good time in a good cause. There was a small organization called the American Woman's Party, headed by Mrs. Oliver Belmont, which used some few of these methods here. It still goes on, in fact, agitating for complete equality between men and women, all the way from the privilege of serving on juries to the elimination of laws protecting women, going so far as to repudiate even maternity legislation. But the bulk of the suffrage movement in this country, thanks to the sound strategical wisdom of Mrs. Carrie Chapman Catt, was just as dignified as it was successful.

When we finally saw the famous Mrs. Pankhurst, she failed completely to be the brawny, rowdy Amazon she should have been. I was on the platform when she addressed a big meeting at Carnegie Hall, so I had a fine look at her—a timid-appearing little mouse of an elderly lady, dressed in Quakerish gray, very tired, very mild, just the type for the vicar's wife in an English village. If this was one of the most dynamic personalities of the time, and that is an accurate description of Mrs. Pankhurst's reputation, something was wrong with my eyesight. She moved wearily to the edge of the platform and began to talk to her packed house of fire-breathing suffrage-enthusiasts as gently and dully as if she had really been the vicar's wife discussing the distribution of soup and flannel to the poor. For the first half-hour she chose to discuss the English governmental system, not a lively subject at best and practically unintelligible to most Americans even if it were exciting. I felt, and could tell that the rest of the committee felt, sick at heart.

Yet it was curiously true that, dull as the content of her speech was and mousy as her manner might seem, she was holding the attention of those thousands of women, even those in the rear of the hall who may well have been having trouble hearing. Then she swung into what we had been waiting to hear—suffrage—and from then on, it was a triumph. Her queer, clear little voice picked up an edge from somewhere and went cutting into the farthest corners of the hall, her little figure straightened and quivered and strained and in no time they were cheering and applauding so frequently that she had to pause between sentences. We did not agree with her methods, but we went away feeling that we had been in touch with an inspired and courageous leader.

Naturally we had to do more than just listen to speeches and attend luncheons and try to get the vote for women merely by holding that thought in the most ladylike manner possible. There was a good deal of fairly unconventional activity connected with our crusading, particularly in the speechmaking department. Few of us reached the high point attained by Inez Milholland, who used to make women's rights' speeches at Poughkeepsie to the Vassar girls. The college authorities would not let her hold meetings on the campus, so she discovered and made use of an old cemetery near by, where the young women used to listen to impassioned outpourings about the wrongs of their sex while seated on cherub-carved tombstones. But any of us who served time as stump-speakers in the suffrage cause got plenty of rough and tumble of the verbal variety to keep things from being too decorous.

You drove out in a wagon or car, pulled up at the curb

on Columbus Circle or Union Square, and stood up and harangued anybody you could get to listen to you. Or else the committee rented a vacant store for an impromptu hall. I did a lot of my orating in such a vacant store on Nassau Street, where we could count on audiences of Wall Street clerks, office-boys and messengers, all killing time during their lunch-hours and looking for amusement. I seldom lacked an audience—an audience exclusively male, average age about twenty-eight, full of scorn for the weaker sex and by no means shy of showing it.

In other words they were natural hecklers and you had to know how to handle them. "Why aren't you home where you belong?" "Who's going to mind the baby when you're out voting?" "Women don't want to vote—it's just the old maids!"—those are fair samples. To listen to them you would have thought every woman in the country who ever stepped out the door of her house was wantonly neglecting three pairs of ailing twins. And I never could make out just how that fitted their conviction that all suffragettes were meddlesome old maids. A ready tongue in your head, giving them as good as they sent with all possible good humor, was the only solution. I was a little shy and mumbly about it at first, but these Wall Street skeptics gave me plenty of experience in a short time and presently I enjoyed myself standing there on a rickety staging and throwing out the answers as fast as the questions came. I never reached the heights of Christabel Pankhurst's classic comeback when she was making a suffrage speech in London. A man shouted at her: "If you were my wife, I'd give you poison!" "If I were your wife," shouted Christabel at the man, "I'd take it!" But I managed the purpose in hand.

For instance, one noontime a fairly bright-looking man

asked me this one, a sample of the occasional intelligent questions: "You say that women will abolish child-labor if they get the vote. All right, women have always had the vote in Wyoming and yet Wyoming has no child-labor law. How do you make that out?" I was pretty well primed with facts and figures, but this one had escaped me. I could afford only a couple of seconds to reflect in, but that was enough: "There are no factories in Wyoming," I said, "so there is no child labor. Wyoming has no child-labor law for the same reason that Massachusetts has no prairie-dog law." A comeback no wittier than that would often bring down the house and get them all on my side. That was the main job—showing them that suffragettes were not window-smashing, bloomers-wearing freaks, but normal, give-and-take people able to take care of themselves and look the world squarely in the eye. We had to have that sort of recognition in order ever to make any headway against the masculine conviction that suffragism was just crank-stuff.

The climax of the campaign for this all-important prestige came in the White House. I had the luck to be there. Up to that point nobody really knew—although there was any amount of wild guessing going on in both camps— just what President Wilson thought about equal suffrage. One evening I received a telephone call from Mrs. Norman Whitehouse, the brilliant field-general of the New York State suffrage army, telling me that she had managed to get the President's consent to receive a small group of prominent suffrage-workers and tell them what his attitude was. She wanted to know if I would be one of the party. I should like to have seen anything that could have stopped me! The committee severally made a dash for Washington trains, rendezvoused at a hotel in Washington the next morning and went in a tense, silent group to the White House.

No one had to say this was a crisis. With the President's prestige on our side, nothing could stop us. With the President against us, or merely passive—that did not bear thinking about. I had not had that exact feeling since the time I marched into the room to deliver my first obstetrical case.

Although this was early in the war, Mr. Wilson was already a tired man; you could see that in his eyes. But he was totally unlike the cold, silent stand-offish person we had been led to expect. There was cordial warmth in his handshake and in his courteous insistence on making us aware that he knew who each of us was and on asking about our personal activities. Then he said:

"I would like to make a speech to the whole group with a stenographer to take it down. I wish I could go and address a large meeting in New York but affairs here will not let me. This will have to be my contribution."

That sounded promising; how promising we did not know until he began to speak. He could not have made a more satisfactory speech if he had asked us beforehand to write down just what we wanted him to say and worked up his speech from those notes. When he had finished, he said:

"Will that do? Will that be of use to you?"

We said that it was several degrees better than perfect and he smiled, then made a farewell round of the group and went out. It was stunning in both the correct and the slang senses of the word.

Largely by accident, I suppose, he had delayed taking a definite stand about suffrage until the exact moment when the psychological effect of his support would do the most good. As we went back to New York we all felt that our

fight had finally been won there in that White House re-
ception room. We were right. At the next election New
York State gave the vote to its millions of women and in a
relatively short time after that the Nineteenth Amendment
was ratified into the Constitution by the thirty-sixth state.

That was at once a great victory and a great deprivation.
When the enemy was routed, the woman's suffrage army
disbanded and we lost all that sense of solidarity and com-
radeship which I valued all the more, I suppose, because I
came into it later than those of my contemporaries who
were among its pioneers. There is no suffrage Grand Army
of the Republic to keep the old campaigners together; we
are scattered, and the vote is won, and the present generation, rightly enough perhaps, doesn't care why, when or
how.

I do not think anyone who was a member of that army,
however, can fail to be bitterly disappointed in the negligible consequences of giving women the vote. I should dislike to try to maintain the thesis that, since the Nineteenth
Amendment was passed, political corruption has been on
the downgrade in American states and municipalities, or
in the Federal government either. And the very fact that
the child-labor amendment is still so far from ratification
should be enough to show how American women have
failed to keep the promises of banding together to improve
social and political conditions which were sown broadcast
as women's suffrage propaganda. I have shouted those
promises myself at street-corner audiences. There is no
such thing as a women's vote that has to be taken into account with the same care as the American Legion vote and
the C.I.O. vote and the farmers' vote; and yet, if women
had really tried to do what they promised to do, their ob-
jectives would probably bear closer scrutiny than those of

any bloc of franchises now cluttering up the American political scene.

It is particularly distressing to an old warhorse who spent a good deal of time in the thick of the suffrage-battle to see that when women do hold office, it is usually as an expedient sop to the female voter rather than because the lady-holder has done the party any large service or because she is extraordinarily good at this job. The number of female office-holders in proportion to the number of men is probably an accurate index of the politician's neglect of the sex that was going to change the world with ballots. Outside politics, boom times put many and many a woman into a man's job, but the depression swept most of them out again. The only place they have held their own is down the scale, where low salaries and no particular need for intelligence keep the economic pressure at lower levels.

Not long ago I went to Washington to attend a dinner of state-directors of Federal child-welfare work. Fifteen years ago, when those jobs were first established by the administration of the Sheppard-Towner Act, only three out of forty-eight of these state-directors were men. Today three-quarters of them are men. I am not impugning the capacity of any of those men as individuals when I say that that looks very strange in a line of activity which was invented and developed by women.

CHAPTER XI

BABIES, WARTIME DOINGS AND MILITANT SUF-
frage work—you can see why I look back on those times
as miraculously full of excitement and dashings to and fro,
no matter how little some of it may have proved effective.
Fortunately for my nervous system, just before the war
broke out, largely against my will, I was forced to abandon
my private practice. For, all the time I had been organizing
the Bureau of Child Hygiene and inventing new ways to
take care of children and fighting for the Bureau's political
life, I had also been carrying on a growing medical career
—largely with children as patients. Neither the organization and development of a new field of public-health activity nor the practice of pediatrics is exactly a part-time
job. It occurs to me now that that may have been why I
never had time for vacations, as other people seem to have.

Or to be exact I had three, two-week vacations during
the first seven years I spent in the Health Department.
Since the summer was the height of our baby-saving campaign, I could never take even those meager holidays when
they were conventionally supposed to come. Instead I
worked at the Bureau night after night. I was actually
enthusiastic enough to be glad that my private practice
tapered off to practically nothing during the summer, so I
could devote myself entirely to the Bureau. I seldom
reached home at night without a briefcase full of papers
for which there had been no time during the day. In order

to free my mind of all possible detail, I evolved a system of sending postcards to myself which I recommend to anybody else with too many things on his mind. When I wanted to remember to bring something from home to office or do something the first thing in the morning, I wrote and mailed myself a penny postcard from the office, which would then appear with my mail and coffee the next morning. If I thought of something at home which needed doing at the office the next day, a similar postcard was dropped in the box and turned up on my desk. If affairs were very pressing there would be a dozen or fifteen of them neatly stacked in each place.

Spending a summer of hard work in New York is not necessarily intolerable. I have done it often enough to know. Dr. Laighton and I had made enough money to take a house for ourselves, a four-story affair which had been built for Rose Coghlan, the great actress, on a side street off Central Park, much too ornate for our tastes but commodious and strikingly cool in the summertime. Whenever there was any spare time, the Park was there, and there were dozens of cool roof-gardens to while away time in. At that time New York was a great center for summer tourists, out-of-towners equipped with guidebooks and umbrellas, earnestly trooping round to see the sights and bombarding bus drivers with questions about everything from Grant's Tomb to the Aquarium. They were harmless and cheery people, and a bus ride among a group of them was as amusing a way to spend the cool evening as anything you can imagine.

No doubt I was still quite young enough to be flexible about things. I could never feel any alarm at all, for instance, about the first car Dr. Laighton and I bought in 1900, with the excuse that it would be useful for calling

on patients; actually, of course, because we were childishly amused with the idea of a new toy. It was a Prescott
steamer, and as cantankerous and cross-grained a contraption as ever rode on wheels. Its water supply would last
only twenty miles, so it was necessary to carry a collapsible
rubber bucket to replenish the supply every hour or so. It
took a good half hour to get steam up in it, once the boiler
was allowed to cool down, which meant unconscionable
delay every time we used it to make calls on patients. Motor
cars were still so rare that, every time we left it at the curb,
we would return to find it completely invisible under a
mass of crawling, prying contemptuous small boys who,
when sent packing, would stand around and hoot, "Get a
horse! Get a horse!" after us as we slowly steamed away.
Public attention was not merely embarrassing. The heating apparatus was a gasoline-spray, which would shoot
flames in all directions as we started up, and every now
and again some excited spectator would turn in a fire-
alarm. No doubt there was a certain truth in the spectator's hasty conclusion that anything which looked that
dangerous probably was dangerous. The interior of the
boxlike thing we sat on, which contained the engine, was
a seething mass of flame all the time. But I could never
worry at all about this intimate contact with potential ex-
plosions. Subsequent cars were probably most unsafe too:
that one-cylindered Cadillac we had, and an Oldsmobile
that steered with a front lever, not to mention two or
three electrics. But the only cars that I have ever managed
to worry about have been the modern highly efficient and
practically fool-proof variety. I suppose that sort of thing
just has to happen to your mental habits as you get older.

Somehow real danger is always hard to believe in. While
I was still in private practice, a woman came to me during

office hours one day and told me she was pregnant, which she demonstrably was, and asked me to sign a paper giving it as my professional opinion that the father of the baby was a certain man from whom she was planning to get money. When I explained that no doctor on earth could conscientiously make such a statement about any baby, born or unborn, she flew into an insane rage and began shrieking that she was going to kill me if I did not sign the paper. That went on for some time, after which I ejected her from the premises with as much dignity as could be managed and went about my business, mildly amused, distressed but by no means inclined to be alarmed. The next day in the paper, I saw a story about this woman. She had made the same proposition to a doctor on Madison Avenue and, when he refused as I had, took out a gun and killed him.

There was hardly more sense of reality about the occasion when a woman shot and killed a man in my Department of Health office. Dr. Royall H. Willis, the Assistant Director of the Bureau, and I were discussing some departmental problem when we heard two shots crash out in the outer office. We ran outside and I saw, without feeling anywhere near as much shock as I should have, a woman standing there with a revolver in her hand, smoke still oozing out of its muzzle, and a man lying face down on the floor, obviously dead. I went up to the woman and held out my hand for the revolver. She gave it to me without any fuss and then we called the police. When investigated, it proved to be the usual story of seduction under promise of marriage. They had had a baby and he had brought mother and child to our office to arrange to have the child boarded out with a foster-mother. The mother, unable to stand the idea of seeing her child taken away, had brought along a revolver and, when the baby was handed over, shot her man in the back, cleanly drilling his heart the first shot. Her second shot buried itself in the wall just six inches over the head of Miss Wilhelmina Rothermund, the Bureau's invaluable Superintendent of Nurses. It was first-degree murder, certainly as deliberate as any crime ever committed. But, after we had talked to the Assistant District Attorney in charge of the case, he agreed to accept a plea of guilty of manslaughter. The man was a thoroughly bad lot who had several other achievements of this sort in his past. The woman had only to serve three years in a reformatory and, best of all, was allowed to have her baby with her while she was there.

There was far more sense of peril in the crisis that arose in my affairs when the question of my Civil Service standing broke over my head in the early part of 1914. With the inauguration of John Purroy Mitchel, who had been elected in the teeth of bitter Tammany opposition, his whole new administration set vigorously to work cleaning up and regularizing all city departments. Our bureau did not need cleaning up. But when Dr. S. S. Goldwater, the new Commissioner of Health, took office, it turned out that regularizing was another matter.

Dr. Goldwater was the finest Commissioner I ever served under, and I served under several very good men indeed. At the time, however, my admiration for him was considerably tempered by the fact that, as soon as he became Commissioner of Health, he insisted that I give up my private practice and concentrate wholly on the work of the Bureau. That was a difficult decision to face. I found that, when I was told I would have to give up my private patients or resign, I liked private practice and would miss it. Besides, it had developed to a point where it was bringing in an excellent income. To confine myself to the Bureau, even at a promised increase in salary, would be a definite financial sacrifice. Once upon a time I had been able to get along on very little income very cheerfully. But it is one thing to start out on a minimum basis and feel merely amused by privations; it is quite another to have worked up mildly luxurious habits and tastes and then have to cut them down. Still, if it was a question of resigning from my beloved Bureau, I had no choice whatever. I could no more have given up that job of my own free will than I could have grown wings and flown. So I sent cards to all of my patients, announcing my retirement from practice, and from then on public health work was the sole reason for my existence.

That had been decided when regularization began in earnest. I found, or rather others found for me, that although I had been regularly promoted by the Board of Health in the past, I had never taken the Civil Service examinations to correspond to my promotions. The first examination, away back in the early days, was my only claim to civil service standing, and that was not enough. The prospect of an examination had never occurred to me, I was much too busy with other things. And it had never occurred to anyone else. So it was made very plain that all of us who had progressed from lowly beginnings would have to take examinations to entitle us to our present jobs. What was worse for me, the examination was open to doctors in lower grades and, if someone earned a better rating than I could, I would be demoted from my position as head of the Bureau. I had everything to lose on the hazard of the examination, and an examination is always a hazard. Everyone else had something potentially to gain. But there was no help for it, and it was a very hot summer, with the battle to keep the baby death rate down always to be waged. The examination, when it came, was the most difficult one I had ever encountered. Both oral and written, the written part lasting a whole day and the oral conducted by a board of New York's best pediatricians.

In September I knew my fate. It was all right. I had passed highest with a grade of 94. My nearest competitor had an 86. At that point I did take a short vacation—fled to the country and took long breaths of undisguised relief. My job was safe—safer than it had been planned to be to begin with.

I was certainly a fine administrator. If it hadn't been for political grudges, I would have gone right through my whole career with the Bureau on an irregular basis and so perhaps robbed myself of the pension that I would receive after twenty years of service. Every time I draw my pension, I think with a tender smile of the way they did me that financial favor in spite of myself.

I doubt if anybody would have tried any such stunt if they had realized how tenaciously I had become attached to my job. I did not realize that myself until, in 1920, I was taken up on a high mountain and shown all the kingdoms of the welfare-earth if only I would leave the Bureau. The tempter in question was that great pair of philanthropists, Mr. and Mrs. Cyrus McCormick of Chicago. They invited me to lunch at the Plaza and told me that the Director of the McCormick Memorial Foundation, a great child-health institution, had been forced to resign and they wanted me to take his place. Money no object: I could have any salary I named; I could direct the Foundation into any activity I pleased; all I would have to do would be to take the Foundation's millions and make them count. An extremely flattering offer and very graciously made. My only answer was, I am afraid, completely bewildering to them:

"I'm sorry," I said, over and over, "but I don't want to live in Chicago . . . I'm sorry. I don't want to live in Chicago."

And that was just it. I did not and do not have anything in particular against Chicago. But I had fought my way through so many battles, private and public, in New York; I knew so much about what lay beneath its harsh, shapeless exterior; I was so much in love with what I was doing, that to consider leaving it was like considering an operation that would completely change my personality. The McCormicks looked more and more puzzled at each repetition of my unwillingness to live in their home town. For several years they kept at me, with their ideas of my salary growing to such fantastic heights that my Health Department salary sounded like the contents of a baby's bank. But, since it was not money I was worrying about, money did not change my mind. I was probably the first thing that McCormick money had not been able to buy, which, no doubt, added considerably to the mystery of my refusal.

No sooner had I retired from private practice than, for my sins, I found myself starting on a career of speechmaking that is not quite over yet and has taken me into every sizable town in the United States. I asked for it in a way. The only method conceivable of putting over the child-hygiene idea with the nation at large was to stand upon my feet and talk about it as often as possible; so that was just what I did. I have trouped as much as an oldtime theatrical star, I think, only, instead of being allowed to arrive in town, put on my act and move on without extra bother, I have always had to be entertained by the well intentioned committee or club that sponsored my speech.

In no time I was sympathizing deeply with Jane Addams' system of charging for lectures. (I suspect it was wishful thinking and not actual practice.) Miss Addams told me once that her charges were on a sliding scale, depending upon what was expected of her: $100 if all she had to do was talk; $150 if she had not only to talk, but to have dinner with someone; and $200 if she not only had to have dinner but to spend the night at someone's house as well. There is no more miserable feeling in the world than to arrive in some average-sized town where you do not know a soul, be met by a collection of clubwomen, dragged to a local mansion for dinner with a lot of people you never want to see again, transported to a stuffy hall to make a speech that you have made a dozen times before and that, to judge from the reactions of the audience, nobody particularly wants to hear—and then, when the one thing that would set you right would be a quiet, empty, private hotel room, be kidnapped after the speech and sentenced to an overnight stay in somebody's cold-sheeted and stiffly furnished guest-room.

I went through years of peripatetic speech-making, however, without realizing that sometimes the hospitable ladies in the towns I visited might feel much the same way about entertaining visiting celebrities. That came out in Utica finally. When the invitation to speak there arrived, it included the usual suave notification that I would be suitably dined and slept. I was in a state of rebellion by then and wrote back that under no circumstances would I put anyone to such trouble; I would go to a hotel and look after myself. When I made my speech, it was received with incredible enthusiasm. You would have thought I was Edmund Burke crossed with Patrick Henry. I could not understand it until afterward, when the ladies of the committee drove me out to a country club. The head of the committee then broke down and explained my popularity. She said that, on dispatching the invitation, she had, as usual, asked the assembled committee who would volunteer to entertain me. I was the last of a long line of the season's speakers, and there was dead silence. Eventually one woman spoke up rather shamefacedly and said that, since she had not yet taken care of any of the speakers, she supposed she would have to. Then the question of who would give a dinner for me: an even longer silence this time, broken by the offer of a lady to assume that burden, accompanied by a heavy sigh. My letter refusing hospitality altogether was a bombshell of joy to them. I could have talked about political economy among earth-worms and they still would have loved me and cheered themselves hoarse for me.

"Why, my dear," said the president, "it's made you the most popular speaker that ever came to Utica."

That is only a sample. My years of speechmaking have been a tissue of absurdities, I am afraid, or perhaps it is just that I have the kind of memory which hangs on to the absurd and forgets things better worth remembering. Chairmen—more frequently chairwomen—used apparently to go out of their way to amuse me. Twice I have spoken at serious meetings to which I was introduced, not as Dr. S. Josephine Baker, head of the New York City Bureau of Child Hygiene, but as Josephine Daskam Bacon, the author. There was nothing to do on either occasion but plunge right ahead and try to behave as if I were Josephine Daskam Bacon, so I did my best, but I have always been afraid that my *alter ego* would sue me for libel any day. I have also been introduced as Dr. Josephine Hemingway Kenyon on occasion, and, back when both she and I were writing for women's magazines, used to get much of her mail. I have had an august chairwoman at a large luncheon turn to me and whisper deferentially:

"Will you speak now, Dr. Baker, or shall I let them enjoy themselves a little longer?"

The effect was often as if the speaker's subject-matter and contributions to it were not the point at all. It was rather as if having any speaker to listen to and applaud afterward were the only essential thing. On one occasion that came out with uncomfortable clarity. The first speaker was a statuesque lady with flowing robes whose subject, according to the program, was to be "In Paradise with Dante." I was somewhat appalled by the idea of getting up and going into the ramifications of anything so practical and sometimes messy as child hygiene after that preliminary. I was even more appalled during the hour that the lady took to soar and swoop through Paradise in such distinguished company. At the end the ladies in the audience all spatted their neatly gloved hands together politely and then all eyes turned to me. I got up and mentally threw away the speech I had prepared. Now that we had been through Paradise with Dante, I was going to take them through Hell's Kitchen with S. Josephine Baker. Purposely, with malice aforethought, I dug out of my memory the most filthy, most horrible, most excruciating details of public health work in general and child welfare in particular and laid them before my audience in the most graphic language I could muster. I went into backyard privies, the fate of stray animals, the worst cases in public hospitals, working hard. Throughout they all gazed at me with the same mild serenity with which they had listened to my aestheticizing predecessor. And, when I had finished, they all spatted their gloves together in exactly the same way and got up, chattering, to have tea. In fact afterward several of them took occasion to tell me how fortunate they had been to have two such interesting speakers the same afternoon. But the essential absurdity of the whole performance never came out more brilliantly than on the occasion when I was to talk to a large convention of public health authorities in Washington on the same program as Jane Addams and many another famous woman. I showed Miss Addams the schedule of speakers:

"Will you please look at this?" I said. "Here they have me down to talk on 'Health—an International Problem.' Twenty minutes. How in heaven's name can anybody say anything worth listening to on that subject in twenty minutes?"

Miss Addams looked at me strangely—I could not tell whether it was a sob or a smile that she was choking down. Then she ran her finger on down the list to this item:

"Jane Addams, 'How to Feed the World,' twenty minutes."

"My dear," she said, "how would you like to try to feed the world in twenty minutes instead?"

Still that kind of memory has its compensations. There was that huge child welfare dinner in Los Angeles given in my honor, where I was the eleventh speaker on the list. Knowing that it was a child welfare gathering, I had prepared, and gave, a speech about child welfare. I give you my word I was the only speaker who came within a mile of the subject. The others were far more eloquent and forceful than I, but Los Angeles, its beauties, past, present and future, were all they talked about, and they seemed to take it unkindly that I had not followed suit. Then there was that other medical dinner out West where I asked a local doctor how he accounted for the fact that, although

Colorado and Utah were right next door and living conditions were practically the same in both states, the Utah maternal mortality rate was so much lower than Colorado's.

"Well," he said, "I do have a theory. After all, any woman who would have followed Brigham Young to Salt Lake City was probably the type that has a good broad pelvis."

I could not get away from the queer things that happened if I tried to make a speech, not even when I went back to Poughkeepsie to address the Vassar girls on the necessity for the modern woman's learning about and following the teachings of modern child welfare findings. At Vassar I was naturally under the sponsorship of Dr. Elizabeth Thalberg, a grand old lady who had been medical director of the college from time immemorial, and whom I had always known just as I had known my aunts and uncles. I have already recorded my own disappointment at having been prevented from going to Vassar. Dr. Thalberg's disappointment must have been even greater than mine because, in the course of my annual lectures, she eventually had both herself and the students convinced that I was as much a Vassar graduate as any real alumna in the world. I started out, accurately enough, as a woman with strong Vassar traditions in her background who had had to give up the idea of going to the college through no intention of her own. In a couple of years, according to Dr. Thalberg, I had matriculated and gone brilliantly into my junior year, when circumstances beyond my control had forced me to withdraw. In three or four years more I had graduated with honors and gone on into medical school with every professor on the faculty looking after me and shaking his or her head and saying: "That girl will make us proud of her, mark my words." It was done so gradually and yet so completely that Dr. Thalberg would have been outraged, I am sure, if anybody had pointed out to her that unfortunately the name of Sara Josephine Baker was missing from the college records. As for myself, I never tried to undeceive her. She got too much innocent joy out of the idea that I was a Vassar girl and, to tell you the truth, I was rather pleased myself with having received a degree without working for it at all.

CHAPTER XII

NEARLY EVERYONE WHO GOES TO RUSSIA ON A
preordained tour rushes into print about it all, at about
the time he steps off the gangplank in New York. It has
taken me four years to succumb to the temptation to write
about what I saw and experienced in the Soviet Union. If I
were not writing about my own past, which includes so
much child welfare work, I might well have resisted to
the bitter end. But the Soviet Union presents the modern
world's most outstanding example of a widespread, comprehensive, centralized system of child welfare and, since
I did see that system in its fairly advanced stages, my
impressions of it definitely belong here. If travel in Russia
were not such an ordeal, I should like to go back to see it
again in a few years to discover how much they have accomplished toward filling the gaps in their practice.

I had not thought of a trip to Russia as a possibility.
But when my friend Miss I. A. R. Wylie told me that she
was going to spend several months there, observing the
Soviet Union in a search for material for a book she was
planning to write, and asked me to go with her, the opportunity seemed one that could not be resisted, and I did
not have to be asked twice. Being aware that strange complaints attacked one in that country, that there is nothing
more dismal than being ill in a strange land without a
doctor of your own kind and that Russian pharmacy supplies were probably not extensive, I started a medicine kit

of my own devising containing remedies for almost every kind of emergency; starting at the top of the head and ending at the toes. Hectic as the trip often was, I never regretted any of it, least of all the medicines in my little bag.

There was a fearful amount of being rubbed the wrong way about the trip, even traveling as we did, first class at from twenty-five to thirty dollars a day each with the extras counted in. We had a special guide and theoretically special accommodations. Actually the accommodations were about the same as those given the second- and third-class travelers—there were "classes" in this presumably Communistic country. But everywhere outside of Moscow and Leningrad there was only one hotel open for tourists and the first party that arrived secured the best rooms, no matter what class they had paid for, and we took what was left if we came later. The car arrangements were probably the most flagrant annoyances. Our rate was to include a Lincoln car wherever we went—Fords and Lincolns were about the only cars in Russia. Often we had one, but there were occasions when the tourist authorities blandly asked us to believe that any car with a motor that would still turn over—or no car at all—was a satisfactory fulfilling of their obligations. Down in the Caucasus, the promised Lincoln turned out to be a nameless mechanism at least twenty years old, a gasping, wheezing, rattling, brakeless outrage, in which we drove over the dangerous stretches of the Georgian Military Highway. The trip was really not so dangerous in itself but it was a characteristic mountain road, narrow and hairpin-turned, where you wanted a car with plenty of power and immediate response to accelerator and steering-gear. When we stopped for lunch, on one of the highest passes, Ida Wylie and I casually looked at this wreck and found one of the rear wheels just in the act of falling off. The chauffeur seemed to take it as a piece of bourgeois insolence that we had found out something it was not our business to know. But he forgave us for meddling sufficiently to put it back on again with a couple of spare bolts and hope. So on we went, but the thought of that wheel somehow prevented my full enjoyment of the scenery.

When we went from Rostov to Ordzhonikidze, the train we were supposed to take was commandeered by a party of high officials on a mission of state and there was an amazing mixup that finally landed us in a desolate town called Minerali Vodi at four o'clock in the morning, tired and rebellious. Our guide, who was one of the nicest boys I have ever known, made a sortie through the town and finally obtained some eggs and a loaf of bread for us. Until noon, we sat in that railroad station and wondered what might happen next. A train arrived. The guide reported that it was absolutely packed. But by that time despair had made me stern and decided. "Ernest," I said, "we are going on that train. It may be on the steps or the roof but that is the train we are going on."

That galvanized him into frenzied action. It happened to be one of the few Russian trains that carried a dining car, so he finally secured us permission to ride in that. It was filthy and full of flies but it did transport us to Ordzhonikidze. When we arrived there with the faint hope that there might be a Lincoln, there was only one car in sight, standing empty in front of the station. We started for this car. The driver spoke sharply to us, explaining that he was waiting for an important official party. I asked where our car was and was told this was the only car in town. So again we sat on the railroad platform. After two hours of waiting, Miss Wylie and I walked over to the car, sat down resolutely in the back seat and waited for the next move. Ernest begged us not to do anything so rash. But we were foreigners and women and, talk as he might, the chauffeur was afraid to eject us, and on we went. I hope the high officials did not have to walk; it was a good many miles and a bad road.

I know many people who have been to Russia and who have never met a bedbug. Why they were kept for us I do not know. Anyway, it was a fairly constant companionship. We had no defense against vermin, but we were careful about diet. No black bread, no uncooked fruits or vegetables and only bottled water. On the Volga, Ernest commandeered a cook, a waiter and special food, and so for that four days we had the best food on our trip. At Stalingrad we left on a twenty-four-hour train trip. It was an 1850 train which in its best moments could make fifteen miles per hour. We were in a compartment with two dingy berths and were told no windows could be opened. It was a hot night in August and that night when we could turn our attention from the bedbugs, we were conscious of the most filthy smell I have ever encountered. In the morning we opened the door and rushed out into the corridor to breathe again and then Ernest appeared ready for breakfast. The mystery of the smell was solved as he reached over our heads into the rack and produced a very inky newspaper package, unwrapped it and brought to view a piece of cold greasy pork, a mass of disintegrated caviar and the most peculiar chicken I have ever seen. It was a brownish purple and had a high gloss on it as though it had been varnished. There was no doubt about the source of the smell and there was no doubt that *we* were going to breakfast on tea alone. But Ernest ate this filthy, inky food. I

[219]

watched him with a horrid fascination, wondering what I had with me that would be an antidote for ptomaine poisoning. I could have spared myself any worry. Ernest was a true Soviet citizen; he stayed in the best of health.

On first thought it seems strange that the Soviet Union should have created so thorough and far-reaching a system of child welfare. On second thought, however, one can see at least two good reasons why it would do this. First, there is the paradoxical sentimentalism of the Russian people. On the one hand, they are extraordinarily brutal in their treatment of their own. The world has had its fill of the horrors of premeditated starvation of huge groups, of "purges" which seem incomprehensible to us, of cold-hearted, bestial brutality and of total indifference to the sanctity of human liberty and life. But there seems to be another side to the Russian character. They are astonishingly soft-hearted and sentimental about anything and everything that has to do with children. Not that this tells the whole story. I have a strong suspicion that the Soviet Government is keenly alive to the necessity of a high birth-rate and the equal necessity of strong and vigorous childhood. Man power for future war material is also a necessity.

During this trip I heard a story which illustrates this strange dual temperament. It concerned an official in high authority in the old Cheka, which was the secret police organization that preceded the famous OGPU. This official had a particular passion for interviewing suspects who had already been made prisoners. His technique consisted of summoning these prisoners, one by one, to his office and listening, with apparent sympathy, to all they had to say. When they were dismissed and started for the door leading out of his office, he would pick up a revolver, which

had lain concealed under some papers on his desk, and,
quite calmly, shoot them in the back. After a morning
spent in that edifying occupation, he would wander over to
the near-by day nursery, which he had founded, and spend
a refreshing half-hour playing gaily and solicitously with
the children there. They told me about him at the day
nursery, but only about this side of his life. And there is
no reason to suppose that, being Russian, he could see or
feel anything incongruous about this startling combination of tastes.

Now the Soviet Union is certainly feeling the full effect
of the demand for child welfare that always arises in any
nation that is frantically preparing for war. It is just another example of the grisly connection between the need
for life and preparation for wholesale death. For its first
ten years, before the policy of fostering the world revolution was officially soft-pedalled, the Soviet Union was
morally certain that the Capitalistic powers would invade
her at any moment. Today, with the ascendancy of Fascist
powers in Germany and Italy and the emerging Fascism
that has always been latent in Japan, war seems even more
imminent than it did in Trotzky's time from the Red Russian point of view. I am far from being an international
political expert but I do know that you could not talk to
any Intourist guide for ten minutes without hearing something about the Red Army and impending war and, from
sickening experience, I know it is no accident that, in
1934, the two groups of Russians who looked really well
fed were the soldiers and the children.

It was exciting for me who had spent twenty-three years
fighting and intriguing to keep a huge municipality interested in babies, compromising here and there and gaining a little as the years went by, to see a whole nation

straining every nerve to give babies and little children the best available, even if it was not altogether the best possible. But there was disappointment too in seeing the inefficiency and the primitive arrangements that, except in the cream of the day nurseries and hospitals, were all too often balking well-intentioned efforts in the Soviet Union. After all, the revolution left little enough of the middle-class Russian medical faculty. Red medicine was woefully short-handed, and, in building up a new generation of doctors, the Communist government had to work far too rapidly to get first-class results in either plant or personnel. It was very hard to find out much about those early, hastily organized medical colleges. But any well-trained doctor is perfectly aware that it takes years and years to build up an institution capable of affording a good medical education and that training ill-prepared young people in a hurry is always a mistake, even in a well-organized and well-staffed medical school. It is probably fair to say that, for some time, a young Russian man or woman could call himself or herself a doctor and be considered fit for practice on the basis of an amount of medical training that, in the United States, would be considered hardly sufficient for a hospital orderly. Nowadays, however, the standard is being raised. No doubt the present standard of medical training would be acceptable in almost every country.

Besides, the profession of medicine was, in those days, competing for the best young blood. Other kinds of technicians—engineers for instance—received much higher salaries than doctors and were likely to attract the more ambitious and possibly more intelligent class of young men. One result of this that naturally pleased me, of course, was that since so many of the better class of young men were crowded into engineering, the bright young

women flocked to medicine. Already in 1928, according
to the figures issued by the state, half of the doctors in
the Soviet Union were women. The proportion continued
to rise until, when we were there, it was quoted at a little
over three-quarters for women. Since doctors' salaries have
recently been put in the same class as engineers' salaries,
the proportions between the sexes in medicine will probably revert to a more even basis. But in view of the impression I often encounter, among people who know Russians well, that the gray mare is usually the better horse,
that may not necessarily be a good thing for Russian medicine. From my own experience I can offer tribute to the
high-minded selfless ambition and professional alertness
of women who are now doctors in Russia.

In acquainting myself with Russian medical standards,
I naturally used American standards for comparison.
Again and again I have been told that this is a great mistake and that the only fair thing to do is to make a comparison with what Russia had *before* the revolution. But
I do not know much about what Russia had before the
revolution and I do know what a reasonable attention to
the dictates of modern medical discoveries calls for in a
modern hospital, whether in America or in the Andaman
Islands.

I think it was the swarms of flies in the hospitals and
day nurseries that bothered me the most. They did not
seem to bother the doctors or the patients or the children.
But it was summer and fairly hot and the best screening
that offered, when there was any at all, was rather decrepit
and often torn mosquito-netting. It was not a matter of
being far from home, unable to understand alien methods;
in Helsingfors, for example, only overnight from the
Soviet border, there were hospitals that, I could see at a

glance, compared most favorably with the best I have ever seen in any city in the United States. So I must go on record here as feeling that the best managed and the best equipped hospital that I saw in Russia—and I saw most of the best hospitals west of the Urals—would be considered third-rate in the United States. Even the nurses, although probably willing enough, appeared barely better than the average ward maid in discipline and training. But you could not convey this impression to any of the modern Russians. One and all, from director down to the least important nurse, they were convinced that the Soviet Union had the finest hospitals, the best doctors and the most widely distributed medical service in the whole world. It was that way with everything. They are all trained to believe that only the Russian brand of Communism can produce any good and there is no point in trying to convince them that the capitalistic world ever so much as heard of a free clinic or a children's playground. I soon learned that no one there had the slightest desire to hear of anything being done elsewhere. If I ventured to suggest that we had ambulances (which they seemed to think they had invented) or that our hospitals offered something that they had not yet heard of, a curious mental blankness would come over their faces; it was as though a screen had been pulled down in front of them. They knew nothing of the outside world and they did not want to know anything about it.

Still, that attitude has produced some fine achievements and some excellent work; they have the spirit of pioneers. There is no reason to believe that they will stop until their system of state medicine and child welfare really is as extensive and as efficient as they think it is now. In fact, if they have, by this time, caught up with their theories, they may well now have the best nation-wide system of child care in the world. But there is a big "if."

I always mistrust people who make broad generalizations about other countries. But I am fairly sure that I made out one significant Russian trait in my contacts with Soviet medical and welfare workers. They seemed to me practically incapable of distinguishing between the honest intention to do something and actually having done it. The idea was just as good as the fulfillment and less trouble. Everywhere we went, for instance, in child clinics and maternity wards there were posters tacked up on the walls, cleverly illustrating the idea that children should get plenty of spinach and orange juice. So they should, and this was extremely well done propaganda. But, unhappily, green vegetables and citrus fruits were practically unobtainable in the whole northern half of European Russia. If you asked: "But where do you get the oranges and spinach?" they would answer: "They are indeed difficult to get," and go on to talk about something else.

Yet no one but me seemed disturbed by the unbridgeable gap between theory and performance. In Moscow I saw the most intelligent educational exhibit of infant hygiene that I have ever encountered. The whole story was there in pictures, models and charts, from conception to school age, covering diet, exercise, mental development, prenatal care, even birth control and abortion. In many other places I saw highly intelligent and effective displays teaching the best birth-control methods. Yet birth control equipment was practically impossible for the mass of the population to procure.

Nevertheless, there was always a counterbalancing, sanguine point of view to cheer you up when these absurdities had depressed you. Those clinics and day nurseries were often astoundingly primitive, but at least they were there, where they had never been before, battering away at superstition and ignorance. In a certain day nursery outside of Kharkov, that has always stayed in my mind as the dirtiest nursery I ever saw, all the little children had to eat was corn on the cob. But that was better than nothing and the state was supplying it free and, if some baby grew sick, there was a sort of doctor in the village, certainly far better than the oldtime herb doctor. Anyone who had been through all I had in the early struggles for saving babies, could hardly be discouraged by the sight of primitive conditions. And, as the least thing you can do for little children is always helpful, so these children were thriving on what was probably the first attempt at adequate care Russian children, as a whole, had ever had. The striking thing in the Soviet Union from the point of view of the child-welfare worker is that, however scrawny and stunted the middle-aged people may look, the youngsters are husky and plump; they look well-nourished and sturdy. And evidently quite smart. Almost universally, children under two years of age could dress and undress themselves with ease. I have seen that demonstrated, at the word of command, many times. In the better nurseries they wore aprons with symbols such as animals or flowers and these same symbols appeared on their mugs and face-cloths. The children could pick out their mugs and cloths at once even as our children do. They told me they had invented this idea and who am I to know better with the pictures of our well-equipped day nurseries in my mind?

The children, however, were dismayingly solemn. That used to worry me an unconscionable amount. It still worries me as I think back to it. If this was just "company manners," then Russian children are the most easily trained of any in the world. I must have seen thousands of Soviet infants and children and, when they were not engaged dutifully in some kind of organized play, they just sat and looked at you like so many little Buddhas. They even had an exact moment when they all sat on their little chamber pots and, to judge by the rest of the system, I could only suppose that their bowel movements were regulated in true Soviet fashion. They never smiled. They never fought. Elsewhere in the world I have yet to see a sizable collection of two- or three-year-olds that will not at some time, in some way, start some sort of disagreement or row, whether there is a visiting foreigner there or not. I found myself actually itching to do something that would startle them out of their abnormal, stolid passivity. For they did not even cry. After you have seen thousands of babies and never even heard a whimper, there has to be a question. "Don't they ever cry?" I asked. "It isn't normal." "No, no," said our guide, rather pleased than not by the inquiry. "Why should a Soviet baby cry? There is nothing to cry about."

That strange placidity seemed to hold good throughout childhood. I bought and brought home several delightful pictures of Soviet children grinning broadly, even laughing, or looking as though they were laughing. But throughout the length of European Russia, from Leningrad to Tiflis, I never saw any laughing children. That sort of thing depresses you just as Leningrad depresses you. In Rostov, way down south not far from the Black Sea, there was a certain amount of movement and gaiety on the streets, a sense of well-being and of having time to be cheerful. But in Leningrad the broad squares and wide streets that the Russian Emperors built to glorify themselves were lined with shuffling, stooping, gray-faced people all apparently walking nowhere in particular, glum, discouraged and pretty sordidly clothed. It seemed to me like a city of ghosts. Throughout Russia there were no generalizations that would hold good. The gray discouragement of Leningrad was, to a degree, offset by the semblance of crowded gaiety of Moscow. The tired, filthy and often diseased condition of the vast storms of people in the little towns along the Volga had its antithesis in the picturesque, astrakhan-capped brigands of the Caucasus. Everything is true about Soviet Russia and, equally nothing is true about Soviet Russia. So I well understand the widely varying stories that can come out of that astonishing land. We were, perhaps, fortunate as we were not on any conducted tour. Just the two of us with our guide who was an ex-Red-Army man and a most delightful companion. He spoke English perfectly, he was young and gay and, above all, constantly solicitous about his "two ladies." Once outside of Moscow and Leningrad where the path is set for all tourists, we were free to go and to see anything we chose. In all we traveled about 6,000 miles. We had gay days and happy ones; we had experiences which still make me shudder. Bedbugs and cockroaches are not desirable bedfellows. But it was a colorful experience.

One thing that depressed me was the rapid turnover in responsible posts, if the medical and child-welfare end of the government is any example. Before we left America and while we were in London, I was well supplied with letters to the heads of the Health Departments of all the Soviets. Some of these came from an eminent Soviet diplomat. By the time we reached the various Soviets, not one of these men could be found. The office was always there but when I asked for the official to whom my letter was addressed, I met a simply evasive reply. "Doctor So-and-so has gone." "No, we do not know where he is." "We will take care of you." I can only surmise that they had all been dismissed from their jobs in the space of two or three weeks and departed to that realm where "purged" Russians lose their names if not their lives. Maybe I landed in the middle of one of the "purges." I do not know; I only know that it did rather alarm me.

I should have been far more puzzled by the discrepancy between the calibre of Soviet sanitation and the healthiness of Soviet children if I had not acquired so profound a respect for the congenital resistance to bacteria of the modern generation of Russians. Ernest's acceptance of that unspeakable meal was nothing unusual. They are evidently immune to practically anything, even a joke. I can only suppose that the non-resistant strains died out during the revolution and the privations that followed and in the succeeding "terrors" of various kinds. We seldom saw elderly people, and few enough that were middle-aged. The streets, theatres and trains were full of people below thirty-five. In fact, Russia is generally populated by a post-war generation, all bred and fed on early hardships. Today, babies are fed solid and horrible food at an age that would frighten an American pediatrician, and they flourish on this diet. Babies can be born and spend their first few weeks in a hospital swarming with flies and yet bid defiance to intestinal diseases. Families and their children can live in insanitary conditions and on a diet that would mean pestilence in this country. And all of them have a stoicism to pain that makes me marvel.

There are two incidents that I remember about this reaction to pain. They could be duplicated all over Russia. One day I was talking to a doctor and asked about his wife. He said she had gone to a dentist to have an impacted wis-

dom tooth pulled. "I hope the doctor has some anaesthetic,"
I said. "Certainly not," he replied. "Why should she have
an anaesthetic? It will not hurt her at all." On another
occasion I was watching one of those famous (and then
not prohibited) abortions. The surroundings were simple;
only a few elementary instruments were used and aseptic
precautions were startlingly lacking, but the technique was
very good indeed. There was no anaesthetic either. No
doctor who has had any experience with gynaecology need
be told that a thorough curettage can cause almost unbearable pain. Yet that woman lay there on the table without
contracting a muscle of her face and without any signs of
distress whatsoever. Toward the end she reached out and
squeezed her nurse's hand a little and smiled. She had been
completely stolid and immobile throughout. Once again I
had to marvel at something I could not believe. "Good
Lord," I said, "how can she keep from screaming?" "Why
should she scream?" asked the guide at my elbow. "She
has confidence in her doctor." The idea that confidence in
the doctor was a substitute for ether was new to me. So
was the fact, as evidenced in Soviet statistics about the results of free public abortions, that to perform curettage
under startlingly insanitary conditions does not necessarily
lead to a high death rate—if the patients are Russians.
The average, as they gave it to me, was one death in every
25,000 operations and the ratio of sepsis somewhere
around .03 percent. The only way I could account for it
was that the Communist Party had outlawed sepsis along
with private ownership of the means of production.

These free abortion clinics were a tremendous storm
center of controversy in the bourgeois world three or four
years ago. They told me in Russia that, in the absence of
effective birth-control equipment, free abortion was the

only solution for the problem of reconciling motherhood with the free status of Communist women. If the state had not performed abortions, they would have been performed privately by Heaven knows who, as they had been before the revolution, with disastrous results. I took the figures they gave me, as to results, with a grain of salt. But after visiting ward after ward of abortion patients with no sign of illness among them all, I was forced to believe in spite of myself.

I admired the Russians' willingness to meet that situation frankly and openly. All doctors know of the deplorable conditions existing in this country. Underground, bootleg abortion is almost always disastrous. And so, I felt a corresponding amount of disappointment when I learned, as the whole world now knows, that the Soviet government has reversed that policy and now prohibits abortion except in the exceptional instances covered by conventional medical reasons. They are in a good strategic position for I can believe there are no doctors in Russia who would dare to perform an abortion. In this country we leave it to the quacks and midwives, and thousands of women die because of this policy. I have heard that one reason for the change in the policy of the Soviet government is that too-frequent abortions are undermining the health of Russian womanhood. That is medically acceptable as a reason. But I suspect that the Soviet drive for more and more population, to offset the German threat on the west and the Japanese threat on the east, has a good deal to do with it. It may be additionally a part of the whole tendency to return to bourgeois principles, to the family, differentiated scales of pay and non-progressive education, all of which have been so evident of late in the Soviet Union. Since the practice of medicine is a state function in the Soviet Union, the government may well be able to suppress private abortion, but I shall be surprised if, with human nature as it is, abortion can be efficiently stopped anywhere else.

Anyway, it was a joy to my professional soul to see institutions like the Prophylactarium in Leningrad—at least that part of it which was a large-scale baby clinic. One of their schemes here struck me as particularly clever and I have seen nothing like it in this country. There was no main entrance, or at least no such thing in a conspicuous position. Instead there was a long array of doors along the front of the building, each door leading into a glass-walled cubicle. When a mother and her child entered the cubicle, a doctor appeared from another door leading from the clinic proper, and thus isolated, the child was examined for the possibility of any infectious disease before it was allowed to cross the actual threshold of the building. If any suspicious symptoms were found, isolation was immediately enforced. This calls for hordes of doctors of course. But there *are* hordes of doctors in the Soviet Union. Moreover, the doctors are distributed throughout the country so that no one need ever be without medical care of some sort.

I wish I might have been equally impressed with the quality and amount of medical supplies in the Soviet Union. When we were there—the same situation must still hold to a considerable extent—drugs and chemicals that medical practice elsewhere considers absolutely essential were available only in pathetically limited amounts. That, of course, is why anaesthetics are used only in major operations and then sparingly. In a provincial Torgsin (foreign currency) store, I remember seeing some digitalis on display for sale in the forlorn drug case. Its label was in English and bore the name of a Russian doctor's laboratory in *St. Petersburg*, which, since that name was changed to Petrograd in 1918, meant that the drug was almost twenty years old. Digitalis at that age is about as much use in the treatment of a patient with any abnormal condition of the heart as a drum with a hole in it would be in an orchestra. When, at the end of our trip, both Miss Wylie and I were victims of various complaints due to the fact that we were not Russian and so not immune to bad food and multitudinous insect bites, I wanted to supplement my supply of bicarbonate of soda, surely an innocent drug. To obtain some, I had to persuade a very special doctor to write me a prescription, and even then all I could get was about one teaspoonful. Later, when Ida Wylie was really ill, her doctor and I had to combine our small stocks of drugs to get the ones that were essential. Notwithstanding my admiration for the state medical system, I could not face with any equanimity the thought of a Russian hospital, so after many conferences with the staff at the American Embassy, I finally found a German doctor in Moscow who was independent and confined his practice to the embassies.

He, and my store of castor oil, saved the situation. For, though I appreciate that to a Russian any doctor is better than no doctor, I doubted if the patient's effete bourgeois constitution could have survived the methods of the local talent.

And yet, the doctors whom we met were delightful people. They were wonderfully cordial and eager to show you all they were doing and all they had with a naïve insistence that, whether it was an X-ray machine or a hypodermic syringe, there was nothing like it anywhere else in the world. I often found it difficult to sit quietly through their long-winded explanations because few of them spoke English and the guides were not often qualified to interpret

and give a detailed explanation of fifteen solid minutes of
a lecture on some fine point of procedure. Once, in that
fine cottage-hospital in Rostov, which I think is the most
modern and probably the best hospital that I saw, I was
hysterically reminded of the "he said yes" business in the
old vaudeville acts I used to see at Proctor's 23rd Street
Theatre in my student days. I was consulting with the
director and his closest associates. They spoke no English
and all the Russian I knew consisted of isolated words—a
hundred or so, few of which were to the purpose. We
bowed to one another and then sat solemnly waiting for
something to happen. My guide whispered to me:

"They are waiting for you to ask them a question."

All I could think of at the moment was the old standard
question, the fundamental inquiry in all infant care:

"What is the baby death rate in Rostov?"

That started the flood of words. My guide rose and made
a long speech lasting some ten minutes. Goodness knows
what she said, but it was eloquent and pithy and delivered
with the oratorical flair of a born stump-speaker. When
she had finished, the director arose and proceeded to show
us how a speech should be made. The guide had been a
clever amateur but this was a masterpiece; portentous,
grave, lightened with flashes of wit, enlivened with homely
philosophy and profoundly stimulating. I could sense all
that by the close attention, the laughter and the solemn
faces of the listeners. Then he bowed and sat down. I
turned to the guide:

"What did you ask him?"

"I asked what was the baby death rate."

"And what did he say?"

"He says it is one hundred and thirty-five."

When we were able to travel, we started for Leningrad

with Elizabeth Embler and Rachel Barrett who had joined us in the latter part of our travels. For a long time neither I nor the embassies' doctor was at all sure that Miss Wylie would ever travel anywhere again, but in some way we did get on that train for Leningrad and there, for a final touch, occurred one of the interesting sidelights on the Communist regime. At the hotel we were given two small rooms over the kitchen, dark, smelly and most uninviting. With my last burst of American surety, I went to the office:

"Surely, you have better rooms than these," I said.

"Nothing better," the clerk replied with finality.

"What about a suite I happened to see on the second floor? You know we are in the first-class category."

Strangely enough he succumbed at once. Producing a key he ushered us into a suite which I am sure must have been reserved for the elite of the land. Seven rooms all remarkably and elegantly furnished with furniture which I am sure came from places of grandeur. It was as Jimmy Durante has said, "colossal, magnificent, almost mediocre!" At any rate, our last days were spent in a burst of glory.

I have never had such a feeling of "Thank God, that's over," as when our train passed over the bridge that marks the Finnish border. Just across a tiny brook from the Soviet Union, it was a different world. With its cleanliness, cheap hotel rates, green forests and glistening lakes, Finland seemed to me to be the loveliest place in the world. I want to go back some day and see if it is really as altogether lovely and cheerful as it seemed to me then, or if it was just the effect of the Soviet Union.

For I came out of Russia in an extremely curious state of mind. Did I, or did I not, believe in state medicine? Did

I know whether to ascribe to the Russian race the strange quirks in temperament I had witnessed or were they to be thought of as part of the Communistic state of mind? As someone who had carved an adequate and personally satisfactory career out of state medicine—for in the last analysis, child welfare in public agencies is merely the most obvious branch of state preventive medicine—I could not help feeling deeply gratified at the spectacle of a great nation really trying, for the first time in history, to make health the privilege of every citizen.

State medicine is to my mind an ideal, and the sooner it changes from an ideal to a practical reality, the better off the human race will be. The mere fact that in Russia every pregnant woman is given ample time off from her work both before and after her confinement and that she not only receives full pay for this time but also has the best care available during her entire pregnancy and confinement, all without cost, means an untold amount to the veteran welfare-worker. I have, perhaps unwittingly, done my share to bring state medicine into existence. I am reasonably certain that the next generation will see it immeasurably advanced in the United States and, unlike so many of my colleagues, I am on the whole pleased with the prospect. It may come about through some form of co-operative plan; it may be the form of "panel system" that seems to work with success in England, or it may be in some other still unthought-of form. It is already on its way and it is now too late for any backward step.

I can quite appreciate the position of organized medicine in its abhorrence toward anything that may interfere with the present isolated integrity of the medical profession. Yet the practice of medicine holds its present status only by virtue of state control. No one can deny that the really poor and, above all, the small salaried class are now facing insurmountable difficulties in obtaining adequate medical care at a price at all within their power to pay. The present cost of medical care is far beyond the capacity of the majority of the citizens of this country. On the other hand, doctors must and should be able to earn a livelihood. State medicine will provide for both sides.

There will have to be safeguards and concessions to our democratic ideals. For instance, when I am ill I want to be free to choose my own doctor. I do not want a doctor arbitrarily forced upon me by the State. But I am convinced that intelligent legislation can meet this difficulty. As far as Russia is concerned I am equally convinced that there was no choice in the matter. It was state medicine or a continuance of the chaotic neglect of the vast majority of the people left over from the old regime. The failures in the Russian experiment need not discourage us. They are the result of the Russian temperament and the Russian history. They are not an inherent feature of the experiment itself. In any case a civilization which insists upon compulsory education must logically insist upon compulsory health of the children it educates.

In general I left Russia feeling that however interesting and exciting the country's social adventures might be, it offered neither an example nor a warning to our more advanced civilization. In fact, at the time of my visit, I could not see that it was an example of any sort. I went to Russia expecting to find a Communistic country; instead I found a form of state socialism almost verging on state capitalism. I went expecting to see equal pay and equal methods of life and living; instead I found as great a hiatus between the rich and the poor as may be found in any capitalistic state. In Russia the poor are still poor and working for inadequate wages; the well-to-do and powerful are, in relative terms, as well fed and housed and as strong in their might as in any other country. And yet, among the masses of the people there was a genuine joy in the thought that they were building a new world on a new basis.

So that my feeling about Russia still remains in a state of something approaching confusion, which recent news from the Soviet Union has done nothing to dispel. The Russians I met were courteous, friendly and charming. They were frightened, it is true; there is fear stalking everywhere in Russia. But I left with an astonishingly friendly attitude toward the place and its aspirations. This sounds fantastic. Even with all the bad mixed with the good, it is so. A book might be written about it all but I am still on the negative side about that. By now, I can say only that it was an inspiring three months—one of the most interesting experiences of a most interesting life.

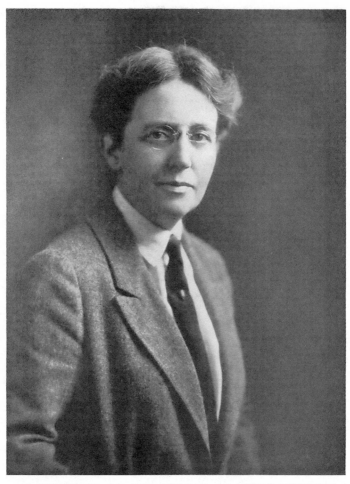

AS DIRECTOR OF THE BUREAU OF CHILD HYGIENE

CHAPTER XIII

In WRITING AN AUTOBIOGRAPHY, ONE HAS THE great advantage of occupying the center of the stage. It is much the same feeling that came over me during those long years when I taught. I knew then that sitting on the right side of the table made an immense difference. It seemed to me to be the real secret of effectiveness in teaching or lecturing. For that brief moment you are there to be listened to, and in a sense, your word is law. When you step down from the platform or out of the classroom, you become a mere mortal again. But meanwhile the advantage is all on your side and the only defense your audience can have is not to listen. So now, I assume the right to give my reactions to my life as I have lived it, and, if they seem pontifical, they can very easily be skipped.

Why do we give birth to and raise children? That question came up very naturally in the course of a career devoted to child hygiene. Frankly, as the years went by, I grew more and more confused about it. Years ago, when the work for saving babies started, there was little or no doubt in my mind that it was a great humanitarian project and that no effort, no matter how great, could be counted wasted if it accomplished this purpose. Not that I was ever even mildly sentimental about working for and with children. There were many times when it seemed quite clear to me that I might as well have been of any business that involved mass production. It brought into

[239]

play all of the administrative and executive functions that might be applied to any large business. Once in a while, it seemed actually necessary for me to make trips throughout the city and to visit the baby health stations and the schools so that the necessary human touch would come back to me. On the whole, my work was strangely impersonal; simply an intriguing proposition that had enough difficulties to make it worth doing. I never gave a great deal of thought to its ultimate purpose. Here was a great waste: my problem was how to prevent it.

Since my ideas and my work have now passed over to many other minds and hands, there has been time for reflection as to its value. I know that any mother and father will think this question has only one answer; they would be shocked even to think that there could be a suspicion that the lives and welfare of their children are not the most important thing in the world. There has never been a doubt in my mind either that, from the family point of view, the safety and well-being of that family's children is of the first importance. Of course it is. The human race is the only species, so far as I know, that has an abiding faith in mother-love—a valuable part of our heritage which we could not efface even if we would. With its protective and holding instinct, it is unique, and although there are many individual tragedies connected with it when it is too much prolonged, its earlier manifestation is one of the finest aspects of family life. In the earliest years of human life, I could ask for even more, and not less, "mothering." It may mean the difference between life and death for a baby. But all this is after the babies come. It does not necessarily play a part in the question as to whether they are worth having or not.

Whatever the answer or the reason, fewer babies are

being born. Several years ago, when I was writing a
monthly article on baby and child care for *The Ladies'
Home Journal*, the continued trend toward a lower birth
rate was becoming manifest not only in this country but
throughout the civilized world. I decided to write an article about it for that magazine. In collecting my facts, I
wrote to a large number of the leading obstetricians
throughout the country and asked them if fewer babies
were being born in their neighborhoods and their practices,
and if so, what in their opinion was the cause of this trend
toward smaller families.

I called the article, "The High Cost of Babies," but that
did not cover the entire problem. The replies to my questions were very interesting and informative. In the cities,
among the middle classes, most young married couples
either had no children at all or limited themselves to one.
The reasons they gave were based upon their economic
status. Small living-quarters in apartment hotels or equally
small apartments afforded no room for additions to the
family. Children invariably meant additional rent and that
was a factor of importance. Then our modern high-geared
life seemed to require the ownership of an automobile.
Only too often the choice was between a motor car and a
baby—the initial cost and the upkeep were about the same
—and the toss frequently went to the immediate motor car
rather than to the future baby. In the less privileged classes
the same sort of consideration was creeping in. During my
lifetime the immigrant family of from six to eight children had shrunk to an average of three or four. Restricted
immigration meant no more replenishments of the type of
European which accepted fecundity as a normal condition.
Difficult economic conditions, meaning fewer jobs, made
children a liability instead of an asset. The second and

third generations were coming to accept the American standard.

The more well-to-do and the wealthy families had a somewhat different answer. Here initial cost and upkeep played no part in the size of families. Motor cars were an accepted and little considered part of daily life. But the arguments for small families were even more emphatic. Doctors whose practice was confined almost entirely to the wealthy but who had no point of contact with each other, invariably wrote me that potential fathers and mothers were refusing to bring children into a world which held such an insecure future. It was not for them to bring up their boys to take part in future wars nor their girls to be plunged into the vicissitudes of an uncertain working world.

There are enough exceptions all around us to prove that this is far from a universal state of mind. We still see and meet families that are fairly large. But we also have enough knowledge of childless "families" to give us pause for thought. Certainly the state of the world during the past few years is enough to give us a sympathetic insight into the minds of those who would limit all offspring for purely unselfish reasons. We must have something better than this to offer our future children, or possibly it may be better that they should not be born. In wondering about this tendency toward a lower birth rate, we should not forget that even Germany and Italy, with their desire for larger populations and the incentives they offer toward increased childbearing, have not been successful in inducing their peoples to respond. Russia is more successful. Since free abortion has been discontinued and the dissemination of birth control information limited or altogether stopped, its birth rate is soaring to almost unbelievable heights.

Which brings us to a consideration of the probable outcome of these changes.

A few years ago I submitted to one of our leading monthly magazines an idea for an article on "A Moratorium for Babies." My theory was that women could force the world to abandon war as a national policy if they would simply refuse to bear children until governments came to their senses, or realized that there would be no future soldiers. I thought it would be an interesting and fairly easy topic. The editor was interested, and I started to work it out. The thesis was sound and workable for all the civilized nations, but it led me into some startling conjectures. The inevitable consequence of any such procedure became apparent. Assuming that Europe and America might well respond to the purpose of this crusade, what of India? What of China? And what of all the other so-called backward—but populous—countries of the world? I began to see our birth rate as a matter of world-percentage. Cutting it down, even if by so doing we might make our civilization still more civilized, could easily mean the end of innumerable gains that we have already made, and the dominance of the Orient or some unthought-of race to whom such ideals would mean nothing!

That is as near as I have come to a logical reason for having babies. Certainly it is worth while for us to keep alive and well those children who are already born or who may be born. Our falling birth rate can be met only in this way. That it has been met, in part at least, is to me a cheering sign. That the progress we have made has been through saving the babies we have from sickness and death, rather than through keeping the birth rate high to cover a high mortality, is even more gratifying. It is evidence that we have the means within our power to solve the problem, at least in part, from the humanitarian, sentimental and world progress points of view.

Granted that this work is worth doing and worth doing well, the enormous impetus that is pushing it forward at the present time is a heartening inspiration. Throughout the world today, the importance of child hygiene is accepted. Within the space of thirty years it has, from an isolated instance, grown to almost unbelievable proportions. In the United States there is hardly a township or a village that at the present time has not established some work for the reduction of infant mortality and for preventing ill health during childhood. I know of no other cause that has grown so rapidly. From its beginning in New York City in 1908, it has advanced so that now each one of our forty-eight states has a Bureau of Child Hygiene, and Hawaii, Alaska and Porto Rico have joined with us in the good work. Preventive medicine as a public service has been established from this humble beginning. Public Health Nurses are found everywhere today whereas, thirty years ago, they were employed only in the New York City Department of Health. The basic principles of keeping babies well that began in our limited efforts in New York City are now so well known that few workers in the field have any idea that they have not always existed. It is difficult for me to comprehend that this acceptance has developed from such recent beginnings and that it is now so great. A great honor and opportunity happened to alight on my doorstep years ago, and a greater honor and deeper satisfaction has come to me in its success. Not that it was altogether easy. The idea was good and did not need much pushing but there were long days of political interference, rank discouragement and constant struggle to keep from being submerged. There were too many days when I could have echoed the words of Abraham Lincoln:

"If I were to try and read, much less answer, all the attacks made on me, this shop might as well be closed for any other business. I do the best I can; and I mean to keep on doing so until the end. If the end brings me out all right, what is said against me won't amount to anything. If the end brings me out wrong, ten angels swearing I was right would make no difference."

Sometimes I could have wished it otherwise. In the earliest years it was practically all struggle. There were, no doubt, many mistakes. That seemingly could not be helped. No one liked a woman in an executive job in a city department. Few tried to help. Later, when results began to come, my friends were many and of the right sort. First among them were the pediatricians of the city, although in the very beginning they too had held themselves very much aloof. I owe a large debt of gratitude to Dr. L. Emmett Holt, Dr. Henry Dwight Chapin, Dr. Herbert B. Wilcox, Dr. Ira S. Wile, and many others. Later the obstetricians came to my aid and all cooperated with the Bureau in many helpful ways. I am proud and honored to count them among my friends. No one could have asked for better support than I had among the professional groups. Though we had our differences of opinion, they were loyal and stalwart champions of our common cause.

I presume I have always had the spirit of the pioneer, and at first, had the gay and gorgeous buoyance of youth. Not that I have recognized it; life has been too busy for that. But as I look back over the years, there seem to have been a surprising number of "firsts" in my life. I suspect that was because women were then making an effort to get out of the shadow-land where they had dwelt for so long, and the enormous vitality and strength of youth made almost anything seem possible. I was young and active during the years when women began to be emancipated and to find their place. I remember a remark that Anna Howard Shaw once made to a reporter who came to see her when women had lost their first battle for the vote in New York State. He asked her how it felt to lose. And Dr. Shaw promptly replied: "We haven't lost. How can one lose what one has never had?" We women had never had any position of importance in the world and, during those years at the turn of the century and soon afterward, we had everything to gain. The pioneer aspect of my work—that I could have been the first woman to earn the degree of Doctor of Public Health, the first woman to hold an executive governmental position, the first woman to be appointed in the professional rank in the League of Nations and above all, the first woman (or man for that matter) to act on the idea that preventive medicine in baby and child care was a function of government—seems very strange and unreal now. But it has left me with a special interest in the achievements of my sex. Today women are everywhere in public life. Not that they have made the strides that I had hoped for them thirty years ago. It seemed for a time—certainly after they received the right to vote— as though the way were clear and open before them. For several years, women went constantly forward. Today, there are many signs that they are content with a lower level of attainment. Possibly the economic condition of the world is responsible, but the fact remains.

I know that in the profession of medicine women are still a long way from their goal and, moreover, that they

FIGHTING FOR LIFE

have been losing their higher grade positions and failing
to get anywhere near the "top." Hospitals still do not open
their doors to women in staff positions; clinics still relegate
them to the lower ranks and, on the whole, they have not
held their hardly won gains of twenty, or even fifteen
years ago. There are always exceptions, of course. In the
political field, several women have proved their calibre.
There are a few, a very few, who have reached the highest
rank in the business world. But, on the whole, women still
hold a very minor place in the working and professional
world. We are all aware of men who stand at the very top
in finance and business who might have great difficulty
staying there if it were not for their able and efficient private secretaries—all women. And yet these latter women,
brilliant as they may be, will go no further.

I hold no brief for women as women. There are good
and bad in their ranks. But I have a strong suspicion that
the same holds true for men, and I do not think that many
women have been the success that they might well be. It
is still a man's world. The vote did not bring us either full
emancipation or full opportunity. We still have plenty of
indirect influence but little that is direct. We have made
some gains but we have also suffered many losses. During
the suffrage days I had no great illusion about my sex; I
wanted the vote as a matter of common justice. But I still
believe that women have something to offer this sick world
that men either do not have or have not offered.

It seems to me that women could make a real contribution in the field of medicine. In the course of my lifetime
that profession has, I fear, become less human. The general practitioner is passing. Today, a patient has virtually
to make his own diagnosis of his ailment before knowing
what doctor to choose to treat him. Specialism is rampant

among both men and women doctors, although women, still at a disadvantage in the profession, increase the hazard if they decide to specialize. It is true today, as always, that the general practitioner could care for, with adequate and good results, at least eighty percent of all the ailments of mankind. The need for highly specialized knowledge is not frequent. And yet, general practice is no longer a lucrative calling. Present methods of diagnosis, for all their elaborate technique, leave much to be desired. It is true that the laboratory and the X-ray have added much that is valuable to our knowledge of diagnosis, but in this change of tactics the average doctor has lost much of his basic skill. Thirty years ago, we had to depend upon our sense of touch, sight and hearing to make a diagnosis, and experience developed an alertness that is not completely replaced by routine laboratory reports. Today this simple efficiency is discarded. No one who is ill can escape the exhausting round of diagnostic methods. A friend of mine told me of her experience in this connection and I relate it here, not because it is unusual, but because it is all too common:

My friend had a sharp pain in her head which she suspected was some sort of sinus trouble, and went first to a nose and throat specialist, who told her that a tonsillectomy, an operation to open up the sinus and a series of hypodermic injections would ease her pain. Not satisfied, she went to a doctor who seemed to be the nearest possible approach to a general practitioner. He suspected a brain tumor and advised her to have her teeth X-rayed and, probably, most of them extracted. To confirm his diagnosis, he referred her to a neurologist. The latter sent her to one laboratory after another: X-rays in abundance, basal metabolism tests, blood counts and blood chemistry, gastric contents analyzed, and other tests too numerous to mention. It took five weeks. Her pain had continued all during this time with increasing intensity; she was on the verge of a collapse. She had had no medical treatment; nothing could be done until a diagnosis was made. At last she went back to the doctor. He was seated before a desk covered with reports from all of her various technicians. He said that now he had a clear diagnosis: every report pointed to sinus trouble and his advice was that she go either to Egypt or to Arizona for the winter! This patient was a working woman. Her meagre savings would not be enough to pay for all of the laboratory reports and the doctors' bills. The prescription, so hard come by, was fantastic. Now she has gone into Christian Science and, so far as I know, is completely well.

I believe that this ultra-specialization is one of the reasons that medicine has its back to the wall and state medicine is on its way. It may be more efficient in the long run, but sick people need immediate help, understanding and humanity almost as much as they need highly standardized and efficient practice. The medical profession is mostly composed of high-minded men, but organized medicine as it exists today in the United States has surrounded the profession with too many taboos and too strong a cult for success to allow it to meet the everyday needs of the mass of the people. I have a great sense of pride in my profession. I know it is moving forward. But I regret the road it has chosen to take.

In the technique of caring for children, I know we have made definite and gratifying progress—although in certain details our attitude has almost described a complete circle in the past thirty years. During my first years in the

Department of Health we undertook to change the habits of a vast tenement population. It was not an easy task, but it was clearly necessary. It was understood by all well-informed persons that babies could be fed on nothing but milk, modified for their age and weight, during their entire first year of life. We were very earnest and sure about this. The newspapers loved to publish sad stories about the iniquities of people who *would* give the baby bits of bacon or cabbage from the family dinner table. It was good publicity but it filled us all with horror that it could be so. Sour milk was supposed to be lethal poison—for babies anyway. Nothing but milk, until the first birthday brought the baby to the beginning of the dreaded carrot-spinach regime. Slowly, but surely, we have now got away from these fetishes, and admitted some virtue in the dire practices of the tenement mothers. Today, babies are fed vegetable purees even as early as five months and spinach and carrots are not the vital magic they were once considered. Many doctors today are using types of sour milk such as buttermilk and koumiss for baby feeding; orange juice is being largely supplanted by tomato juice, and we are catching up with the old time mothers.

There was a period when the vitamin idea threatened to undermine the mentality of many young mothers. Vitamin D was poured into and onto babies and young children in such vast amounts that doctors were forced to call a halt. All of us need a proper amount and a proper proportion of all the vitamins. These can be obtained in any well balanced diet; all human need for them can be met in this simple way. There are times when a greater supply of one or the other may be indicated, but not through self-medication. The doctor, and only the doctor, should make the decision about this.

I suppose the hardest lesson a mother can learn is that babies are very simple little folk and that they need very simple care. The fact becomes very clear when you are dealing with them in large numbers. Saving babies—*en masse*—is the easiest job in the world. No one can claim much credit for a successful baby-saving campaign. But it does need common sense. The simpler the procedure for any organized attempt to save babies is, the better the results will be. Because this is so, the greatest chances for success in any such crusade will lie among those families which we call underprivileged and which are certainly poor. Among our well-to-do population babies are too well cared for. The baby death rate, in New York City at least, bears testimony to that fact: it is higher in the "better" districts than it is in the "poorer" ones. There are several reasons for this. One is that over-elaborate care is economically impossible in poor families. Another is that the mothers in the tenement districts are willing to learn: they will follow directions no matter how strange and outlandish they may seem. And then, babies in the less favored part of our population have acquired an immunity toward disease that the well protected baby has little or no chance to obtain. I, for one, should not like to start a baby-saving campaign among the wealthier class. I am sure it would fail. And I am equally sure that I, or anyone else, by following simple rules, could reduce the baby death rate in any town or city and under the worst conditions in the poorer sections.

The same problem can be seen among children of a slightly more advanced age: undernourishment, for instance, is not found among the children of the poor to the extent that it may be found among the children of the rich. In the tenements the cause of undernourishment may be too little food, the wrong kind of feeding, lack of ventilation, bad family conditions or overstimulation. These conditions are not hard to correct among the poor; there are many helping hands held out to supply the obvious need. But among the well-to-do it is not a question of too little food or the wrong kind; it is rather that the superabundance does not tempt the child's appetite. The child who "will not eat" is seldom the child who has not sufficient food. Overstimulation and overexcitement are far more common among the children of the rich than among the children of the poor. A child can be too well-bred to be healthy—and that is a sad commentary upon our civilization.

There is still much work to be done in the field of child hygiene. Every baby can have a chance for life. This cannot be given by the mother and father alone; it needs more help than that. Our goal will be reached only when public health officials, social welfare agencies, doctors, nurses and parents work together. And this is not so difficult as it sounds. We all know how it can be done; we have known it for many years. We simply do not follow the line that will be surely successful.

Because statistics are strange and unreliable things, I do not want to quote them. I have seen strong men so disturbed as to the accuracy of statistics that they have forgotten the facts they represent. I do not want to be led into this blind alley. I am interested in the child and want to keep first in our minds that we are talking about children and not about their representation as fractions. In dealing with children we are not facing a scientific problem which can be measured wholly in percentages. We are dealing with a human group with only one factor in common— that of age. We are dealing with little Susan and John and

Mary and Thomas. They are our children. Each one carries all the potential possibilities of all humanity. Whatever the statistics say, each has a right to live. And each *can* live. We have not yet made that literally true, but in time we can reach this heart-warming goal. Even with conditions as they are today we have come a long way along this road. Millions of children are living today who might have died without organized care. Our baby death rate has gone down, in New York City, from 144 per thousand births to less than 50 per thousand births this last year. During the hot and enervating summers we have seen the baby deaths decrease from fifteen hundred a week to around sixty a week. I expect to live to see the day when any city or town will hide its head in shame if its baby death rate goes over twenty-five per thousand births.

The way is a simple one. In my official lifetime, the baby death rate has been reduced two-thirds, but this reduction has taken place almost entirely in the class of diseases which we call gastro-intestinal. The diarrhoeal diseases have been met and conquered. The old legend of the deadly first summer is now a part of our folklore. If we are to save the babies represented by the present death rate, we must look for other causes to attack. There is one part of the baby death rate that has been static: there are as many babies dying today during the first month of life as there have ever been. This accounts for one-half of all baby deaths. We have done nothing about it—and we could.

We know that this death rate during the first month of life could be reduced by two-thirds almost at once if every pregnant woman could have proper prenatal care. Here is a reform which might be instituted almost overnight. Instead of a few sparsely located prenatal clinics serving an infinitesimal number of our pregnant women, we might have prenatal care demanded as part of the required studies of every medical student; we might have a prenatal clinic in every hospital and we might have organizations like the American Medical Association conducting graduate courses in prenatal care in every community. The Federal Children's Bureau, under the Social Security Act, is already planning for many of these clinics, but this is not enough. Thirty years have elapsed since we first knew we could reduce our infant mortality in this simple way and we are still talking about it. It seems to me that women, as a group, might demand this and see that it is done. I cannot see why prenatal care for every pregnant woman is not a possibility and why it should not be accomplished within the very near future.

There are other problems that still need to be solved. Healthy babies need healthy mothers, before and after birth. Our present death rate of mothers from conditions during pregnancy and confinement is almost the highest of any of the civilized countries of the world. England has a rate one-third lower than ours; the Scandinavian countries have long had a rate two-thirds lower than ours in the United States. It is of little use to say that this is due to our midwives; both England and the Scandinavian countries employ midwives in far greater numbers than we do. This is a problem for organized medicine to solve, though prenatal care will go a long way to help. A special committee of the New York Academy of Medicine in a report a few years ago gave it as their conclusion that seventy-five percent of these deaths from septic infection at the time of child birth are preventable and that sixty-six percent of the total deaths are likewise preventable. And yet we do nothing, or very little, about it.

Another—and very serious—unsolved problem in child

hygiene is the proper care of the pre-school child. And this ties up with the health problem of the child of school age. We have learned to take care of our babies, but when they pass into childhood they are left to fend for themselves to a large extent. This has been called "the neglected age," "the in-between-child age" and many other epithets of a like forsaken character. It is probably the most important age of our entire life cycle. Ninety percent of cases of contagious diseases occur before the child is five years old; nourishment which may make or mar the health throughout life is determined at this time; character and habits are formed, and the entire groundwork for life is laid then.

But before we argue as to what should be done for the pre-school child, let us go on to the next group—the child of school age. "School age" is an arbitrary limitation, but from the physical angle it does seem to mark a turning point. The height of physical hazard has passed by the time a child enters school; the dangerous age is over so far as contagious diseases are concerned, but it is just beginning with regard to physical defects. At the risk of repeating myself, and for all the emphasis I can bring to bear, I want again to say that if we might thoroughly examine each child when he first enters school; have one hundred percent follow-up work with enough home visits by nurses to make this possible and, as nearly as possible one hundred percent corrective treatment for all physical defects found, we could solve the distressing problem of how school medical inspection might be made worth while. If we would concentrate almost all of our time and money upon this important early procedure, the remainder of our work to keep children of school age healthy would be easy indeed. Of course, there would be a few years' interim of seeming neglect of the older children; the same thing happened when we stopped treating sick babies and bent all of our energies toward keeping them well. It is the only solution of the problem that I can see. That it will be done, I doubt. I can only hope.

We first made progress in saving babies when we stopped caring for sick babies and concentrated on keeping the others well. We knew that a few babies might die who otherwise might have had a chance for life, but we also knew that thousands would live in the future because we had the courage to begin at the right place. We have not had that courage in caring for children after infancy. The political angle has been a deterrent: educational authorities concentrating on their particular jurisdiction have called aloud for a physical examination of each school child each year. There has never been and there never will be enough money available to make any such ideal a possibility. It could not, in any event, be the most efficient and sensible procedure. If we would face the problem honestly, we would admit the far greater usefulness of making sure that children are completely healthy when they enter school.

Of course this means extra concentration on the pre-school child. The neglected age should be neglected no longer. These millions which are now being so ineffectually spent on the school child as a matter of routine, would have to be, in large part, spent on the child *before* he enters school. But by doing this we can solve the problem of health for the school child in short order. School inspection for the detection and control of contagious diseases will still be necessary but these diseases have decreased so in their occurrence that this procedure will take very little money.

In recent years the pre-school child has received a fair share of attention from the psychologists. But we have been so absorbed in the field of mental hygiene and the behavior problems of young children that we have almost totally neglected their health and its implications. It may be well to have a well behaved child; it is of greater importance to have a child who *can* be well behaved. We are already in danger of making the bearing and bringing up of children such a complicated process that many women are afraid to undertake it. Children have always been "bad"; they used to be corrected in various old-fashioned ways, and they outlived the badness in a majority of instances. There is more juvenile delinquency today than there was thirty years ago. Ordinary child "badness" was not considered to be a pathological condition then. Nowadays if a child is anything but a little robot he is taken to a child psychologist to have the cause discovered. The net result is that mothers are unduly apprehensive and children are watched so closely that the tension is disastrous for both.

Children are natural exhibitionists. They love to be noticed and they like to hold the center of the stage. We may well be starting toward breeding a race of little prigs, if not worse. A few years ago I received a report from one of the most prominent nursery schools in this country. In it were listed over three hundred actions which mothers were encouraged to observe in their children: whether they started walking with the right or left foot, whether they noticed this or that, all simple and normal actions and of no consequence to the development of the child. The report gave me a mental picture of maniacal mothers and children to match. Overanxiety on the part of mothers is extremely

[257]

bad for children who find themselves the focus of this anxiety. Probably there are children who need this kind of expert care. But I am sure it is overdone and need not be so universally applied as it is today.

It would be most inappropriate to end my story with an account of unsolved problems. Looking back over my experience of thirty years with children I find the good and the bad intermingled in my remembrance. There were small failures but greater successes, heavy handicaps and great opportunities, side by side. For a clearer picture I must compare the beginning and the end. In a recent issue of "The Child," a U. S. Children's Bureau publication, I find encouragement. The infant mortality in the United States in 1936 was 57 per thousand live births. Not as low as it should and could be—but lower by more than half when compared to the rate of thirty years ago. The provisional rates for 1937 show that during that year 2,775 fewer babies died than during 1936—that is the lowest infant death rate in the history of this country and compares favorably with the baby death rate in any country of the world.

We are making gains in maternal mortality too. For so many years we have had a black record here: the only countries which could show a worse one were Chile, Lithuania, Northern Ireland and Australia. In 1936 our maternal mortality rate was 57 per ten thousand live births —the lowest ever recorded in the United States. Still, the rate is 28 deaths to ten thousand live births in Norway, 30 in the Netherlands and in Italy, 32 in the Irish Free State and 33 in Sweden.

There is no adequate reason why we should not equal these figures. We know how. I hope to live to see the day when death from the preventable disorders of the first month of life has been almost completely abolished; when maternal mortality in the United States is as low as human knowledge can make it; when the pre-school child receives the simple care that assures him of a healthy life. All of these things may be accomplished by the use of already available knowledge. It is to be hoped that we will use this knowledge.

I have stood at the corner of Fifth Avenue and Forty-second Street in New York City and watched the crowds pushing and milling back and forth with set expressions and determined faces, all bent on getting somewhere at the cost of the men or women at their elbows. I have stood there and wondered. Wondered deeply and been sadly perplexed. Should we bring more and more babies into this troubled world? Should we try to keep them alive and well? What is to become of them? Are they to be simply more cannon fodder? There is no clear and certain answer. But the occasional discouragement that gives rise to such questions is only a momentary reaction.

I have faith in the ultimate decency of mankind. I believe that this salvaging of human life has been worth while. I can still see the light in a mother's eyes when her baby was assured of health. When I think back over the long years of hard work and struggle, my joy when ideals were realized and my determination to try over again when things were blackest, my loyal friends and co-workers—I come back to the place where I started. Of course I would do it again. I would not have any of it different in any way. It was a magnificent opportunity, a great and heart-warming experience, a happy road to follow. A glorious, an exhilarating and an altogether satisfactory life.

A few months ago I happened to read the following

excerpt from a little booklet called: "So Near the Gods,"
published by the Society of the New York Hospital:

"A child born this year will probably live fourteen years
longer than one born twenty-five years ago. Expectancy
of life has been increased through the prevention of disease and death during the first two years of life. There has
been no greater gift than this in all the history of mankind."

Perhaps this holds the most fitting tribute that I can pay to
everyone, not only in our New York Bureau of Child
Hygiene but to all the thousands of other consecrated workers who have carried on.

INDEX

[261]

TITLES IN SERIES